HEALTH
PLAN

HEALTH PLAN

The Only Practical Solution to the Soaring Cost of Medical Care

ALAIN C. ENTHOVEN
MARRINER S. ECCLES PROFESSOR
Public and Private Management
Stanford University School of Business

ADDISON-WESLEY PUBLISHING COMPANY
Reading, Massachusetts • Menlo Park, California
London • Amsterdam • Don Mills, Ontario • Sydney

Portions of this book first appeared in:

New England Journal of Medicine **298** (March 23, 1978): 650–658; **298** (March 30, 1978): 709–720; **298** (June 1, 1978): 1229–1238. Reprinted by permission from the *New England Journal of Medicine.*

National Journal **2,** 21, May 26, 1979. Reprinted from *National Journal,* the Washington weekly on government affairs.

Harvard Business Review **57,** 1 (January/February 1979). Reprinted by permission of the *Harvard Business Review.* Copyright © 1979 by the President and Fellows of Harvard College; all rights reserved.

Library of Congress Cataloging in Publication Data

Enthoven, Alain C   1930-
  Health plan.

  Includes index.
  1. Medical economics—United States.   2. Insurance, Health—United
States.   3. Medical policy—United States.   I. Title. [DNLM: 1. Costs and cost
analysis.   2. Economics, Medical—United States.   3. Insurance, Health—United States.
W275 AA1 E6h]
RA410.53.E57   338.4'7'36210973   79-25583
ISBN 0-201-03143-4

Second printing, March 1981

Copyright © 1980 by Addison-Wesley Publishing Company, Inc. Philippines copyright
1980 by Addison-Wesley Publishing Company, Inc.

ISBN-0-201-03143-4
ABCDEFGHIJ-DO-8987654321

TO HAROLD B. FENECH, M.D.,
from whom I have learned so much.

ACKNOWLEDGMENTS

This book has received the benefit of
the thought and generosity of many friends and colleagues. A brief ac-
knowledgment here can only begin to express my appreciation and in-
debtedness to them.

Scott Fleming introduced me to the idea of universal health insurance
based on competition in the private sector. He shared with me notes and
memoranda on the subject that he had prepared while serving as Deputy
Assistant Secretary of HEW. His "Structured Competition Within the
Private Sector" was the progenitor of Consumer Choice Health Plan. We
have discussed these ideas often, and I have profited greatly from his
deep insight and extensive knowledge of health care organization and
finance.

Paul Ellwood, M.D., and the talented associates he has drawn to
InterStudy have also been an important source of inspiration and ideas.
His work and that of Walter McClure and Jon Christianson of Interstudy
have been particularly important sources for this book.

I owe a special debt of gratitude to Patricia Drury, my research associate at Stanford. She took my first draft and, with her powers of clear,
well-organized thinking, brought greater clarity of expression, vigor, and
brevity to my presentation of this very complex subject. She contributed
many useful ideas and served as a valuable colleague and untiring worker
through the development of this book.

John Bunker, M.D., contributed a great deal to my understanding of
medical care. Lewis Butler contributed an uncommon degree of common
sense and wisdom to the development of my proposals. Victor Fuchs
contributed more than any other economist to my understanding of the
unusual and complex economics of health care. Walter McNerney was
very helpful with valuable advice and information. Roger Noll collaborated
with me on a paper on regulation in health care and taught me much of
what I know about that subject. (Chapter 6 draws on that collaboration.)

Christiane Jose, my secretary, managed my office, defended my door
and telephone so that I could write, coped with repeated interruptions,
and typed the drafts and the final manuscript. And she did it all with
unusual skill, dedication, and grace.

As well as from most of the above-mentioned, I received many val-
uable criticisms and suggestions on part or all of a draft from David Chin,
M.D., Richard F. Enthoven, Martha Gilmore, Kevin Hickey, Stanley Jones,
Harold Luft, Bruce Sams, Jr., M.D., and Thomas Senter, M.D.

Needless to say, any remaining errors are mine, not theirs, and the judgments in the book are not necessarily in agreement with theirs.

Finally, I would like to thank some of the people who made it possible for me to write this book. Marriner S. Eccles endowed the professorship that I am proud to hold. Arjay Miller, former Dean of the Graduate School of Business at Stanford, attracted me to Stanford and provided much support and encouragement. Joseph Califano took me on as a consultant on national health insurance when he was Secretary of Health, Education, and Welfare. It was in that capacity that I developed Consumer Choice Health Plan. Whatever might be his views on the economic marketplace as a regulator of health care costs, his commitment to the free marketplace of ideas is strong. The Henry J. Kaiser Family Foundation supported my writing and research with a generous grant. And finally, special appreciation goes to my wife, Rosemary, for her encouragement and help and to her and our children for their patient forbearance while I devoted many hours to the book that could have been spent with them.

Stanford, California   A.C.E.
February 1980

CONTENTS

INTRODUCTION AND SUMMARY   xv
THE GROWTH OF HEALTH CARE SPENDING   xv
CAUSES OF INCREASED SPENDING   xvii
THE REAL ANSWER: FUNDAMENTAL REFORM   xxi

CHAPTER 1: WHAT MEDICAL CARE IS AND ISN'T   1
SEVEN MISCONCEPTIONS ABOUT MEDICAL CARE   1
WHY FINANCIAL INCENTIVES MAKE A DIFFERENCE   9
WHY THE CASUALTY INSURANCE MODEL DOESN'T
FIT MEDICAL CARE WELL   10

CHAPTER 2: IRRATIONAL INCENTIVES AND THE
GROWTH OF HEALTH CARE SPENDING   13
THE GROWTH OF HEALTH CARE SPENDING AND
THE CHANGING PATTERN OF FINANCE   13
    Growth of Spending   13
    Changing Sources of Funds   14
    What Is the Problem?   15
MAIN CAUSES OF SPENDING INCREASE   16
    No Rewards for Economy   16
    Growth and Impact of Insurance Coverage   17
    Impact of the Tax Laws   19
    Fee for Service   21
    The Key Role of the Physician   23
    Cost Reimbursement for Hospitals   24
    The Passive Role of Third-Party Payors   25
    More Doctors   24
    Technology   28
    Aging Population   31
    Other Causes   31
ARE DEDUCTIBLES AND COINSURANCE THE
SOLUTION?   32

CHAPTER 3: CUTTING COST WITHOUT CUTTING THE
QUALITY OF CARE   37
REGIONAL CONCENTRATION OF SURGERY AND
OTHER SERVICES   37
    Open-Heart Surgery   37

Maternity 41
Other Services 41
MATCHING RESOURCES USED TO THE NEEDS OF
THE POPULATION SERVED 42
CURTAILING "FLAT-OF-THE-CURVE" MEDICINE 45
Diminishing Marginal Returns Explained 45
Wide Variations in Per Capita Use of Services, with
No Discernible Difference in Health 46
Length of Hospital Stay for Heart Attack Patients 46
Second Opinions for Surgery 47
Electronic Fetal Monitoring 48
The Need for Benefit-Cost Analysis 49
A Consumer- versus Provider-Oriented Concept of
Quality 50
THE CONTROLLED INTRODUCTION OF NEW
TECHNOLOGY 51
SIMPLE COST CONSCIOUSNESS 53
Equivalent Care in Less Costly Sites 53
Duplicate Tests, Excessive Hospital Stays, Sheer
Waste 54

**CHAPTER 4: ALTERNATIVE FINANCING AND DELIVERY
SYSTEMS** 55
THE HMO ACT AND THE IDEA OF ALTERNATIVE
DELIVERY SYSTEMS 55
EXAMPLES OF ALTERNATIVE DELIVERY SYSTEMS 57
Prepaid Group Practice 57
Individual Practice Association 61
Primary Care Network 64
THE SIGNIFICANCE OF ORGANIZED SYSTEMS OF
MEDICAL CARE 67
GOOD HMOs, BAD HMOs, AND THE HMO
UNDERSERVICE ISSUE 68

**CHAPTER 5: ECONOMIC COMPETITION AMONG
HEALTH CARE FINANCING AND DELIVERY SYSTEMS:
PRINCIPLES AND EXPERIENCE** 70
PRINCIPLES OF FAIR ECONOMIC COMPETITION 71
Multiple Choice 71
Fixed Dollar Subsidies 71
Same Rules for All Competitors 72
Doctors in Competing Economic Units 72
CURRENT LACK OF FAIR ECONOMIC COMPETITION
IN HEALTH SERVICES 72
Economic Competition Explained 72

Most People Don't Have Multiple Choice 73
Most People Don't Get Fixed Dollar Subsidies 75
Different Rules for Different Competitors 77
Most Doctors Are Not in Competing Economic Units 77
WHY WE CANNOT HAVE A COMPLETELY FREE
MARKET IN HEALTH INSURANCE 78
"Free Riders" 78
Preferred-Risk Selection 80
Income Distribution 81
Information Cost 81
EXPERIENCE WITH HEALTH PLAN COMPETITION 82
The Federal Employees' Health Benefits Program
(FEHBP) 82
Hawaii 84
Minneapolis–St. Paul 85
Project Health, Multnomah County, Oregon 88
WHAT CAN WE EXPECT FROM THE FAIR ECONOMIC
COMPETITION OF ALTERNATIVE DELIVERY
SYSTEMS? 89

CHAPTER 6: WHY PRICE CONTROLS AND SIMILAR
CONTROLS DON'T REDUCE HEALTH CARE COSTS 93
REGULATION AS A SUBSTITUTE FOR APPROPRIATE
ECONOMIC INCENTIVES 93
PRICE CONTROLS ON HOSPITALS: HOSPITAL-COST
CONTAINMENT 95
HEALTH PLANNING AND CERTIFICATE OF NEED 101
CONTROLS OF PHYSICIANS' FEES 105
UTILIZATION REVIEW AND PROFESSIONAL
STANDARDS REVIEW ORGANIZATIONS 108
REGULATION VERSUS COMPETITION 110

CHAPTER 7: CONSUMER CHOICE HEALTH PLAN 114
BACKGROUND 114
MAIN IDEAS 115
Universal Health Insurance Independent of Job
Status: Consumer-Centered Rather than Job-
Centered Health Insurance 115
Equitable Distribution of Public Funds 117
Reform Through Incentives 118
Make the Market Work 119
Demonstrated Practical Experience 119
THE FINANCING SYSTEM 119
Actuarial Categories and Costs 119
Tax Credits 121

Vouchers for the Poor   123
Medicare   124
Regional Differences   126
CREATING A SOCIALLY DESIRABLE COMPETITION:
CRITERIA FOR QUALIFIED HEALTH PLANS   126
Open Enrollment   127
Community Rating   127
Basic Health Services   127
Premium Rating by Market Area   128
Low Option   128
"Catastrophic Expense Protection"   129
Information Disclosure   129
Health Plan Identification Card   130
FEDERAL-STATE ROLES IN FINANCING AND
ADMINISTRATION   130
SPECIAL CATEGORIES—DEFENSE DEPARTMENT,
VETERANS, INDIANS, MIGRANTS, THE
UNDERWORLD, ILLEGAL ALIENS, NONENROLLERS,
OTHERS   131
Beneficiaries of Public Direct-Care Systems   131
Migrants, Derelicts, the Underworld, Illegal Aliens,
Nonenrollers, Others   131
TRANSITION   132
PUBLIC POLICY TOWARD DELIVERY-SYSTEM
REFORM   133
COSTS AND THE FEDERAL BUDGET   134
CCHP: SOME ISSUES AND ANSWERS   137
Speed of Reorganization   137
"Consumer Choice"   138
Fairness to the Poor   139
Underserved Rural Areas   140
"WHAT'S IN IT FOR ME?"   140
TWO MAJOR PROBLEMS   142
Government as Gatekeeper   142
Discontinuity   144

**CHAPTER 8: STEPS TOWARD COMPREHENSIVE
REFORM**   145
REQUIRE EMPLOYERS TO OFFER EMPLOYEES
CHOICES   145
REQUIRE EQUAL FIXED-DOLLAR EMPLOYER
CONTRIBUTIONS   148
STANDARDS FOR ALL HEALTH-BENEFITS PLANS   149
FREEDOM OF CHOICE IN MEDICARE   150
A LIMIT ON TAX-FREE EMPLOYER CONTRIBUTIONS   150

FAVORABLE RESPONSE FROM KEY MEMBERS OF
CONGRESS   151
FURTHER STEPS   153
CONCLUDING REMARKS   154

APPENDIX: SUMMARY AND ANALYSIS OF OTHER
LEADING NATIONAL HEALTH INSURANCE PROPOSALS   157
THE KENNEDY PLANS   158
    Health Security   158
    Health Care for All Americans   161
MANDATED EMPLOYER-PROVIDED INSURANCE FOR
THE EMPLOYED AND PUBLIC INSURANCE FOR ALL
OTHERS   167
    The Nixon Proposal   167
    The Carter Proposal   168
    Discussion   170
GOVERNMENT AS UNIVERSAL THIRD-PARTY PAYOR   170

NOTES   173

INDEX   183

INTRODUCTION AND SUMMARY

Like most industrialized countries, the United States has a serious problem of rising health care costs. Unlike most countries, however, we have the opportunity to create a unique solution based on rational economic incentives and a carefully designed system of economic competition in the private sector. To seize this opportunity, we must be willing to take a fresh look at the fundamental causes of the problem and at the record of successes and failures of the attempts to solve it. This chapter presents a summary of the analysis set forth in this book.

THE GROWTH OF HEALTH CARE SPENDING

Health care costs are straining the federal budget and the budgets of many state and local governments.

Public-sector spending on health care services increased sevenfold in the thirteen years from 1965 to 1978, from $11 billion to $78 billion.

Total federal outlays for health care services rose from $4 billion in 1965 to a projected $59 billion in 1980. Medicare, the federal health insurance program that was enacted in 1965 for the aged, is about doubling every four years, growing from about $9 billion in 1972 to $18 billion in 1976 and then to $34 billion by 1980. What is new and different now is the sheer size of the outlays. A doubling of 1980's $34 billion will cause much more strain than did doubling 1972's $9 billion.

These costs are on a collision course with growing resentment over both increasing tax burdens and inflation fueled by federal deficits, not to mention pressures for increased public spending for energy and national defense. Government will be forced to act to bring health care spending under control.

Health insurance costs are also straining private employers. General Motors' payments for employee health insurance rose about sevenfold from 1965 to 1977, increasing from $170 million to $1.2 billion. Chrysler's 1979 health insurance cost per active employee was about $2600. Although the auto industry is an extreme case, large increases have also been experienced by companies in other industries. Much of this money could have gone to employees in the form of more pay or other benefits. Health care costs have thus become a burden on insured workers, even when the employer pays the full premium.

At the same time, despite the growth of insurance, health care costs increasingly burden individuals. Private direct payments for personal health services were $101 per person in 1965 and $248 in 1978. This was a 26 percent increase, even after adjusting the 1978 figure for overall inflation in the economy. Government payments for health care services for persons aged sixty-five and over increased from about $133 per capita in the year ending June 1966—the last year before Medicare—to $892 per capita in 1975. Nevertheless, payments for health care services made directly by the aged patients themselves rose from $234 to $390 per capita from 1966 to 1975. This increase is in about the same proportion as that in the consumer price index. Thus health care costs rose so quickly that Medicare did not succeed in reducing the real burden of health care costs on the aged.

In total, the dollars spent on health care in the United States, an amount that was $43 billion, or $217 per capita in 1965, reached $192 billion, or $863 per capita, in 1978. As a fraction of the gross national product, this spending went from 6.2 percent to 9.1 percent. Even after correcting for general inflation, real per capita spending on health care services doubled over these thirteen years.

Despite these large outlays, by 1978 some 5 to 8 percent of all Americans still had no health insurance, public or private. Millions of others had poor or inadequate coverage. Many were unable to buy private coverage, but had incomes too great to be eligible for Medicaid. Medicaid, a federal program administered and partly paid for by the states, does not cover all of the poor.

Have the benefits been worth the cost? Has all this spending yielded a substantial improvement in the health of the American people? We really don't know. Data on life expectancy suggest that there has been some recent improvement. But once a reasonable minimum level of care is provided, factors other than medical care—diet, lifestyle, heredity, environment—appear to have much more effect on health and longevity than does more or less medical care. Above a reasonable minimum, the availability of more medical care resources appears to have little or no effect on many indicators of health status.

Moreover, much of the value of medical care relates to the *quality* of life—to the relief of suffering and the restoration of function. And we have no good statistical tools to measure this on an aggregate basis. So we cannot give a clear answer to the question of whether or not we are getting much health improvement for these large increases in spending.

If people were generally using their own money to buy medical care, one could argue that they must consider the services received to be worth the cost; otherwise, they would not buy those services. But most people are not using their own money directly. Most people have health insurance that pays much of the cost of their care. And in turn their insurance is heavily subsidized, if not provided free, by their employers or the government. Thus the present organization of health care financing, the familiar health insurance system, does not inspire confidence that people are demanding or getting good value for the money spent.

There are problems other than cost in our health services economy. We appear to have too many hospital beds and too much costly specialized equipment. There is concern about uneven geographic distribution of doctors. (However, there is no good reason for supposing that a completely even distribution would be the "right" one.) Overall, we seem to have too many specialists and subspecialists, too few family doctors or other generalists. (However, we have no good standards for evaluating specialty mix.) There does not seem to be any systematic force working to bring about either an even geographic distribution or a matching of beds, equipment, and numbers of specialists to the needs of the people served.

CAUSES OF INCREASED SPENDING

Many factors contribute to the cost increase: general inflation in the economy (though, as we have seen, health spending has grown at more than twice the general inflation rate), better and more widespread insurance coverage, new technology, an aging population, the increase in malpractice litigation, and others. Some contributors have been surprises. In the 1960s we almost doubled the number of students entering our medical schools, only to find in the 1970s that more doctors mean more doctoring and higher fees. Overall, there has been much overuse of services (excessive hospital stays, duplication of tests), overinvestment, and waste.

I believe, however, that the *main cause* of the unnecessary and unjustified increase in costs is the complex of perverse incentives inherent in our predominant system for financing health care. The "fee-for-service," or piecework, system by which we pay doctors rewards the doctor with more revenue for providing more, and more costly, services, whether or not more is necessary or beneficial to the patient. Physician gross incomes account for only about 18 percent of total health care spending (16 percent if the laboratory tests they order are excluded), but physicians control or influence most of the rest. They admit people to the hospital, order tests, and recommend surgery and other costly procedures. Yet our system assigns them very little responsibility for the economic consequences of their decisions. Most physicians have no idea of the costs of the things they order—and no real reason to care.

Hospitals are paid on the basis of either their costs or charges based on costs. The net effect is that more costs mean more revenue. Those who make the decisions concerning the use of hospital services, doctors and insured patients, have no reason to be cost-conscious. Most medical bills are paid for by "third-party payors," insurance companies and government agencies that pay the bills after the care has been given and the costs incurred. And they are powerless to control costs. Most consumers' insurance gives them free choice of doctor and hospital and little or no incentive to seek out a less costly doctor or style of care. Their personal insurance premium will be the same whether they go to the most economical or the most extravagant doctor. This system embodies many cost-increasing incentives and virtually no rewards for economy. The problems of irrational economic incentives in health care are explained in more detail in Chapter 2.

Why have we chosen a financing system with such perverse consequences? The reasons are many and complex. Some are historical accidents. One important factor has been the medical profession's insistence on the principles of *fee-for-service* payment and *"free choice of doctor"* in every insurance plan. Fee for service is advantageous for doctors, both economically and in ensuring their independence. Freedom of choice of doctor is important to doctors and patients. But insurance with "free choice of doctor" effectively rules out economic competition among doctors. The insured patient has little reason to care about medical costs. Medicare and Medicaid were made to conform to these principles.

Other factors have reinforced the system of insured fee for service. In effect, the *tax laws* put the control of health insurance for employees and their families into the hands of employers by making employer contributions to health insurance tax-free. Employers and unions have used this control to make themselves the workers' benefactors. For the most part, they have chosen to offer employees a single health insurance plan with "free choice of doctor" rather than a menu of competing alternative health plans, each associated with a limited set of doctors. All this is not surprising.

What is more surprising is that the rest of us should have accepted this system. I believe that one reason for this is that we have accepted some basic misconceptions about the nature of medical care. Many people seem to think that medical care is like mechanical engineering—that for each medical condition there is a "best treatment," a "professional standard." It is up to the doctor to know that treatment and to use it. People do not fully understand the great uncertainties that pervade medical care and the variety of acceptable treatments. They think of medical care as mostly treatment for acute life-threatening conditions, as if it were accurately represented by the television dramas about the emergency room. Based on these misconceptions, we have applied to medical care a financing system that was developed for casualty (fire and collision) insurance.

The ideal case for casualty insurance is one in which the damage is caused by an act of God and the cost of repair can be determined objectively. In such a case the financial incentives inherent in insurance do not play a significant role in either the incidence of damage or the cost of repair. Insurance of houses against hurricane damage or fires caused by lightning does not bring on more storms. Collision insurance for automobiles fits the model tolerably, but much less well. Most people do not drive less carefully just because they have insurance. But those who do have insurance are likely to demand more and better repairs than those who do not—because someone else is paying the bill. Still, ordinarily, having your collision-damaged car repaired is not an open-ended task.

Medical insurance hardly fits the model at all. The element of judgment and choice in the decision to seek care and in the amount of care provided is too great. Caring for a patient can be open-ended, especially if he or she has a chronic disease. Uncertainty pervades medical diagnosis and treatment. In most cases there is not one correct or standard treatment. There may be several accepted therapies. Most medical care is not a matter of life and death, but rather of darker or lighter shades of grey concerning the quality of life. In view of this, it should not be surprising that the institutional arrangements for providing care, including the financial incentives facing the doctor, are very important. The casualty insurance model does not fit medical care at all well, because making more care free to the patient and remunerative to the doctor leads to more, and more costly, care being demanded and provided. Some of these insights into the nature of medical care are developed in more detail in Chapter 1.

Insured fee for service is not the only way health care can be financed. Successful alternative financing and delivery systems reward doctors and hospital administrators for finding ways to deliver better care at less cost. In these systems participating physicians accept responsibility for providing comprehensive health care services to their enrolled members, usually for a per capita payment set in advance. This gives the providers of care a fixed budget within which they must do the job, rather than an open-ended source of funds. The list of such systems includes prepaid group practices, individual practice associations, and primary care networks.

Many comparison studies show that prepaid group practices reduce total per capita costs of medical care by 10 to 40 percent compared with the costs for similar people cared for under insured fee for service. Such systems now care for millions of people. Some have done so successfully for decades. Their experience suggests that physician organization and incentives are the main keys to health care cost control. These alternative financing and delivery systems are described in Chapter 4.

The experience of alternative delivery systems shows that it is possible to cut cost without cutting the quality of care. We are not confronted by an immutable tradeoff among cost, quality, and access to care. On the contrary, quality and economy often work together. For example, the best and most economical surgeons are likely to be the busy ones. Their medical results are better because they are proficient. Their costs are lower because they can make a good living while charging low fees. Thus one key to economy and quality in medical care is a careful matching of physician personnel and other resources to the needs of the population served. Another key is the avoidance of care that yields no apparent health benefit.

The physicians in the alternative delivery systems tend to hospitalize their patients some 30 to 45 percent less than do doctors working under insured fee for service. These doctors recognize that *more* care is not necessarily *better* care. Cutting cost without cutting the quality of care is the subject of Chapter 3.

Three broad alternative strategies have been proposed for bringing health care costs under control. The first is direct government controls on prices and capacity, based on the model of public-utility regulation. The second is to require insured patients to pay directly an increased share of their medical bills by increasing deductibles and coinsurance. The third is to create a system of fair economic competition among alternative financing and delivery systems in which the successful ones will be those that produce the best value for consumers, including control of costs. In the face of this choice, public policy has been ambivalent. There has, understandably, been little political support for increased coinsurance. Some reasons for this are explained in Chapter 2. In 1973 the federal government took an important procompetitive step by requiring employers to offer their employees the option of joining a health maintenance organization (HMO), if available. But unfortunately, the main direction of public policy in the 1970s has been toward direct controls.

Starting in 1977, the Carter administration sought to enact an annual percentage limit on the growth of hospital spending or hospital cost per case. In effect, this would have been a continuation of the hospital-cost controls applied by the Nixon administration as a part of its Economic Stabilization Program from 1971 to 1974. Several states have enacted hospital rate control programs. The National Health Planning and Resources Development Act of 1974 required the states to enact "certificate-of-need" laws, regulation of hospital capacity executed through local authorities called health systems agencies. At the time of enactment of the national law, about half of the states had such laws.

In 1979 the Carter administration proposed that the Department of Health, Education, and Welfare (DHEW) establish a schedule of physician fees which all doctors serving Medicare and Medicaid patients would be required to accept as payment in full. We get useful clues as to the likely effects of this kind of regulation by examining the experience with physician fee controls in this country under the Nixon administration's Economic Stabilization Program and in Canada under its national health insurance. In 1972 Congress directed DHEW to create Professional Standards Review Organizations, a national system of local physician organizations charged with responsibility for reviewing the appropriateness of hospital use under the Medicare and Medicaid programs. By 1977, roughly half of the designated areas had such organizations functioning.

The main thing wrong with these controls is that they do nothing to correct the existing cost-increasing incentives. In fact, they often reinforce them and create new ones. By accepting present costs and fees as the basis for future allowable increases, they often reward the fat and punish the lean. At best, they are pure spending restraints that, excepting Professional Standards Review Organizations, ignore health care efficiency, quality, and equity. The substantial research literature on these controls is reviewed in Chapter 6.

For the most part, these controls have proved to be ineffective in restraining health care spending. This failure should not be surprising. Medical care has many characteristics that make it particularly unsuitable for successful economic regulation. Because of the nature of the service, the government cannot measure output or evaluate quality (except in cases of extreme abuse). The "doctor office visit" and the "patient bed day" are not standard units whose prices can be regulated like passenger miles or kilowatt-hours.

Some argue that the remedy for the ineffectiveness of these controls is more rigorous regulation, a comprehensive system with firm ceilings on total health services spending. In effect, the government would control the whole health services industry in detail, including the budget of every hospital and the fees of every doctor. Under such controls, health services would resemble a nationalized industry. But recent studies suggest that among the least efficient and least satisfactory health care systems in our country are those run by government agencies such as the Veterans Administration and the Defense Department. The merits of turning the rest of our health care system over to detailed government control are, to say the least, not obvious. Among the worst consequences of such a system of controls would be the freezing of the health services industry in its present wasteful and inequitable patterns. Rigidity is inherent in a system of public-utility regulation.

THE REAL ANSWER: FUNDAMENTAL REFORM

What I believe is needed is not more bureaucratic controls imposed on an inherently irrational system, but rather fundamental reform of the financing and delivery system itself. *That is, we need to change from today's system dominated by cost-increasing incentives to a system in which providers are rewarded for finding ways to give better care at less cost.* Government cannot reorganize the health care system by direct controls. But government can change the tax laws and the Medicare and Medicaid laws that create the underlying incentives. Government can create a system of fair economic competition in which consumers and providers of care, making decisions in an appropriately structured private market, would do the work of reorganization.

I believe that the only way to get such fundamental change is through competition in the private sector in a market that is free enough to allow such changes to happen. In an appropriately designed system of fair economic competition among various types of health plans, including traditional insurance and fee for service as one option, consumers who join health plans that do a good job of controlling costs would pay lower premiums or receive better benefits. Health plans that do a poor job of controlling costs would lose customers and risk being driven out of business. In the long run, the surviving health plans would be the ones that offer a good value to their members. The health care system would be transformed, gradually and voluntarily, from today's system with built-in cost-increasing incentives to a system with built-in incentives for consumer satisfaction and cost control.

The most important principles of such a system of competition are *multiple choice* and *fixed-dollar subsidies*. Once a year, each family (or individual) would have the opportunity to enroll for the coming year in any of the qualified health plans operating in its area. The amount of financial help each family gets toward the purchase of its health plan membership—from Medicare, Medicaid, employer, or tax laws—would be the same whichever plan it chooses. The subsidy might be more for poor than for nonpoor, for old than for young, for families than for individuals, but *not more for people who choose more costly health plans*. The family that chooses a more costly plan would pay the extra cost itself. Thus it would have an incentive to consider the cost. In addition, physicians would be organized in competing economic units (most would participate in one or another alternative delivery system), so that the premium each group charged would reflect its ability to control costs.

The main problems in our health care economy arise from the fact that for the most part, these principles are not applied today. Most people, when they come to work, are presented with a *single* employer-provided health insurance plan. Among those employers that do give their employees a choice, many pay the whole premium either way and thus eliminate the employee's financial incentive to choose the less costly plan. The aged are locked into Medicare, the eligible poor get Medicaid, both based on fee-for-service and cost-reimbursement principles. Thus Medicare, Medicaid, employer, and tax laws systematically pay more on behalf of beneficiaries who choose more costly health care plans or providers. What government and these employers are doing is to assure the more costly providers who work in the system of fee for service and cost reimbursement that there is no need for them to control costs. And they are creating a major barrier to new alternative financing and delivery systems, because one of the main things some of the new systems have to offer is cost control.

There are a few groups and market areas in which the principles of competition have been applied, substantially if not completely. The Federal Employees' Health Benefits Program, in successful operation since 1960 and now serving nearly 10 million people, offers employees a multiple choice of alternative plans and a fixed dollar contribution toward the plan of their choice. California offers state employees a similar choice. (Each has minor exceptions to the equal-dollar-subsidy principle.) These systems provide us with some large-scale and long-standing examples to show that competitive systems are practical and workable.

In the few places where it has been tried, competition has been an effective contributor to cost control. The best examples are Hawaii, where most people belong to either Hawaii Medical Service Association or the Kaiser-Permanente Medical Care Program, and Minneapolis, where seven health maintenance organizations compete. Although other factors contribute to cost control in Hawaii, and competition remains attenuated by various government programs, the two plans compete vigorously, and their premiums for comprehensive care are among the lowest in the country. Hawaii's per capita hospital costs are about two-thirds of the national average, despite the fact that consumer prices generally are 20 percent higher in Hawaii than in the rest of the country.

Health plan competition in Minneapolis is much newer. The decision of major employers to adopt competitive principles is fairly recent. From 1972 through 1979, HMO membership grew at a 28 percent annual compound rate, reaching 300,000 in 1979. On average, these organizations hospitalize their members only about 500 days per 1000 members per year, compared with about 850 days for similar people in the community on fee for service. Hospital costs are a major part of total costs, so reduced hospital use is a key factor in overall cost control. The principles of competition and our experience with their application in health care are reviewed in Chapter 5.

These competitive principles are the basis of my comprehensive national health insurance proposal, called Consumer Choice Health Plan (CCHP). Government would help people enroll in and pay for the private health care financing and delivery plan of their choice with tax credits and vouchers, that is, premium contributions in fixed dollar amounts based on both financial need and predicted medical need. Health plans eligible to receive these payments would have to comply with a system of rules designed to foster socially desirable competition. CCHP is modeled on the Federal Employees' Health Benefits Program and similar nonfederal programs. It would extend to the whole population and to all participating health plans its proven principles of fair economic competition, multiple choice, private underwriting and management, and periodic government-managed open enrollment. CCHP is explained in Chapter 7.

Alternatively, we could apply the same principles in a few low-cost "incremental" measures, small steps that would greatly enhance competition and the performance of our private health care financing system. For example, I have recommended that Congress require employers above a certain size to offer their employees *a choice* of competing health plans and to make their contribution in the form of a fixed dollar payment. These two requirements would not be onerous for employers; some have already adopted them. The same principles could be embodied in a "freedom of choice" provision in Medicare. Today, Medicare beneficiaries are vulnerable to large uncovered expenses. Yet they are not allowed to realize for themselves most of the savings generated by joining an efficient alternative delivery system. The law could be changed to permit any beneficiary to direct that the "adjusted average per capita cost" to Medicare for people in the same actuarial category be paid, as a fixed premium contribution, to the alternative delivery system of his or her choice, provided it meets reasonable federal standards. These and other steps toward a universal system of fair competition are reviewed in Chapter 8. Bills to implement these and similar ideas were introduced in the Congress in 1979.

Would competition produce the desired reforms? Would alternative delivery systems that use resources wisely win in a fair competition and replace insured fee for service? There are good reasons for cautious optimism, provided one is not looking for unrealistic "quick fixes." First, the economic advantage of the best alternative delivery systems is large. Second, health maintenance organizations have done well under conditions of fair economic competition. Third, there already are active alternative delivery systems in many communities, despite the existing disincentives. The idea of alternative financing and delivery plans such as HMOs has achieved enhanced legitimacy in recent years. Blue Cross and Blue Shield are now involved in some sixty-six alternative delivery-system developments. Kaiser-Permanente is finding great acceptance among employers in its new entry into Dallas, in sharp contrast to its new-market entries of a decade ago. Prestigious multispecialty group practices, such as Henry Ford Hospital in Detroit and St. Louis Park Medical Center in Minneapolis, have entered the HMO field. The success of Harvard Community Health Plan in Boston is putting pressure on other groups to form competing health care plans. The Lahey Clinic has stated its intention to do so. The idea is no longer just "California Dreaming."

Alternative delivery systems have been sponsored by many types of institutions. Many potential sponsors exist in most communities. The list includes physician groups, industrial companies, insurance companies, Blue Cross–Blue Shield, unions, universities, consumer cooperatives, and hospitals. Many more would emerge if the economic conditions were favorable.

Competition would not work quickly, and it would not work perfectly. Even if CCHP were enacted, it would take a decade or more before half of the population was cared for by some kind of alternative financing and delivery system. But in an imperfect world, the principles of fair economic competition would at least point the health care system in the right direction—toward organized systems with built-in incentives for economy and consumer satisfaction.

There is now intense debate over the pros and cons of the various regulatory devices. National thinking about health policy is drowning in a welter of complex arguments about the detailed merits of each of the regulatory measures. There is a growing recognition that past regulatory strategies have failed. The overwhelming majority of studies by scholars outside government support that conclusion. Moreover, many of the regulatory devices have an ad hoc character. They are improvised emergency limits on spending and contain little or nothing to improve the quality of services or the equity with which they are distributed. Many proponents of direct controls recognize that they are little more than temporary expedients to hold the line while a longer-term solution is being developed. But we seem to be far from agreement on the character of that solution.

An analysis in greater depth is needed. We need to step back from the battles over the various proposed temporary expedients and look for the fundamental causes of our problems. Public policy needs to be guided by a coherent vision of long-term goals and effective means for moving our health care system toward them. The main purpose of this book is to contribute to that vision.

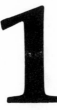

1

What Medical Care Is and Isn't

$\mathbf{M}$ost people think of the need for medical care as an insurable event, very similar to insured hurricane or automobile collision damage. You are either sick or well. If you are sick, you go to the doctor. The doctor diagnoses your illness, applies the standard treatment, and sends the bill for his or her "usual, customary, and reasonable fee," all or most of which is paid by your insurance company. Our entire Blue Cross–Blue Shield and commercial insurance system was built on that view of the problem. Medicare and Medicaid, the public insurance systems for the elderly and poor, were built on the same model. The consequence is a financial disaster. Our society has accepted the casualty insurance model for health care financing, only to find that it contributes to excessive and excessively costly care.

Some people think of medical care as a kind of public utility. It does respond to a vital need, and many people think of it as inherently a monopoly—or at least as unsuitable for competitive private enterprise. As a consequence, we are now in the process of accepting the public-utility model of health care regulation, only to find that it is ineffective. The instruments of public-utility regulation are too blunt to grasp something as variable and imprecise as medical care.

SEVEN MISCONCEPTIONS ABOUT MEDICAL CARE

How is it that models that fit medical care so poorly could be so widely accepted? One reason, I believe, is that many people hold some basic misconceptions about medical care. In order to establish a conceptual framework that fits the realities, we must clear away seven popular misconceptions that underlie the acceptance of these inappropriate models.

1. *"The doctor should be able to know what condition the patient has, be able to answer the patient's questions precisely, and prescribe the right treatment. If the doctor doesn't, that is incompetence or even malpractice."*

Of course, in many cases the diagnosis is clear-cut. But in many others there is a great deal of *uncertainty* in each step of medical care. Doctors are confronted with patients who have symptoms and syndromes, not labels with their diseases. A set of symptoms can be associated with any of several diseases. The chest pains produced by a gall bladder attack and by a heart attack can be confused by excellent doctors. Diagnostic tests are not 100 percent reliable. Consider a young woman with a painless lump in her breast. Is it cancer? There is a significant probability that a breast X-ray (mammogram), will produce a false result; that is, it will say that she does have cancer when she does not, or vice versa. There is less chance of error if a piece of the tissue is removed surgically (biopsy) and examined under a microscope by a pathologist. But even pathologists may reach different conclusions in some cases.

There are often no clear links between treatment and outcome. If a woman is found to have breast cancer, will she be better off if the whole breast and supporting tissue are removed (radical mastectomy), only the breast (simple mastectomy), or only the lump (lumpectomy)? There is considerable disagreement among doctors because there is, in fact, a great deal of uncertainty about the answer. Because of these uncertainties, there is wide variation among doctors in the tests ordered for similar cases and in the treatments prescribed. As Stanford economist Kenneth Arrow observed: "The special economic problems of medical care can be explained as adaptations to the existence of uncertainty in the incidence of disease and in the efficacy of treatment."[1]

2. *"For each medical condition, there is a 'best' treatment. It is up to the doctor to know about that treatment and to use it. Anything else is unnecessary surgery, waste, fraud, or underservice."*

Of course, in many cases there is a clearly indicated treatment. But for many other medical conditions there are *several possible treatments*, each of which is legitimate and associated with different benefits, risks, and costs. Consider a few examples.

A forty-year-old laborer's chronic lower-back pain sometimes requires prolonged bed rest and potent pain medication. One doctor may recommend surgery; another, hoping to avoid the need for surgery, may recommend continued bed rest and traction followed by exercises. Whether one treatment is "better" than the other depends in part on the interpretation of the diagnostic tests (how strong the evidence is of a surgically correctable condition), but also in considerable part on the patient's values and the surgeon's judgment (how large a surgical risk the patient is willing to accept for the predicted likelihood of improvement).

As another common example with more than one treatment, consider a young woman with abnormal uterine bleeding, a nuisance but not a serious health hazard. One doctor may recommend a hysterectomy, whereas a second may advise that a dilatation and curettage be done as the first course of therapy, a third may feel that hormonal treatment is indicated, and a fourth may recommend no treatment. Any of the four might make sense, depending on the circumstances. There is no formula for calculating "the best" treatment, no clear dividing line between a "necessary" and an "unnecessary" operation.

A patient's needs, preferences, and lifestyle are important. Consider a woman who likes to ski and ride horseback and who has a partially detached retina in one eye. One ophthalmologist believes in an operation that does a minimum amount of "welding" (photocoagulation) and would minimize her loss of vision. Although that might satisfy the physician's criterion of technical excellence, it does not allow the woman to resume her athletic pursuits safely. Another ophthalmologist might propose to coagulate a complete circle around her retina. In this case the patient would lose some vision, but would have more of a guarantee that the retina will not detach again, and she could ski and ride again.

Patients suffering from severe angina pectoris (chest pain thought to be due to a lack of oxygen supply to the heart) pose another therapeutic dilemma. One doctor may recommend heart surgery; another, treatment with drugs such as nitroglycerine. For most such patients, there is no consensus among physicians today as to which is the better treatment.

What is "best" in a particular case will depend on the values and needs of the patient, the skills of the doctor, and the other resources available. The quality of the outcome depends a great deal on how the patient feels about it. What is an annoyance for one patient may mean the inability to keep a job for another with the same condition. There is nothing wrong with the fact that doctors disagree. There is plenty of room for honest differences based on these and other factors. There are more and less costly treatments, practice patterns, and styles of medical care that produce substantially equivalent medical outcomes.

Medical care differs in important ways from repair of collision damage to your car. If you have a smashed fender, you can get three bids and make a deal to have it fixed. You can tell when it is fixed. There is one "correct treatment." Ordinarily, it should not be an open-ended task. But caring for a patient can be open-ended, especially when there is a great deal of uncertainty or when the patient has a chronic disease. Walter McClure, an analyst with InterStudy, a leading health policy research institute, put the point effectively when he wrote:

> The medical care system can legitimately absorb every dollar society will give it. If health insurance is expanded without seriously addressing the medical care system itself, cost escalation is likely to be severe and chronic. For example, why provide $50 of tests to be 95% certain of a diagnosis, if $250 of tests will provide 97% certainty.[2]

Although there are generally accepted treatments for many diseases, and doctors can agree that there has been bad care in some cases, for many others there are no generally agreed standards of what is "the best" care. Physicians reject suggestions of what they refer to as "cookbook medicine"; recognizing the infinite variety of conditions, values, and uncertainties, they are understandably reluctant to impose such standards on one another.

The misconception that best-treatment standards exist for most cases underlies much of the belief in the feasibility of an insurance system like Medicare and the hope that regulatory schemes such as Professional Standards Review Organizations can control costs. If we understand that often there is no clear-cut best course of action in medical care, we will think in terms of alternatives, value judgments, and incentives rather than numerical standards.

3. *"Medicine is an exact science. Unlike 50 or 100 years ago, there is now a firm scientific base for what the doctor does. Standard treatments are supported by scientific proof of efficacy."*

In fact, medicine remains more of an art than a science. To be sure, it uses and applies scientific knowledge, and to become a physician, one must have command of a great deal of scientific information. But the application of this knowledge is a matter of judgment.

To prove beyond reasonable doubt that a medical treatment is effective often requires what is called a "randomized clinical trial (RCT)." In an RCT a large sample of patients is assigned randomly to two or more treatment groups. Each group is given one of the alternative treatments and then is evaluated by unbiased observers to see which treatment produced the better results. One of the "treatments" may be no treatment. (Of course, RCTs may not be needed in the case of "clear winners" such as penicillin, treatment of fractures, and congenital anomalies.) However, many practical difficulties stand in the way of doing a satisfactory clinical trial. As a result, RCTs are the exception, not the rule.

When medical or surgical innovations have been evaluated in this way, more often than not the innovation has been found to yield no benefit or even to be inferior to previous methods of treatment.[3] Even when a clinical trial has established the value of a given treatment, judgment must be used in deciding whether a particular patient or set of circumstances is enough like those in the trial that the same good results can be expected in this particular case.

There are shifting opinions in medical care. Many operations have been invented and enjoyed popularity, only to be subsequently discarded when systematic testing failed to demonstrate their value. Benjamin Barnes, M.D., professor of surgery at Tufts University Medical School, provided numerous examples in his history of discarded operations between 1880 and 1942.[4] More recent examples include gastric freezing as a treatment for duodenal ulcer and internal mammary artery ligation as a treatment of angina pectoris.[5] Whether or not the coronary artery bypass graft operation that has recently become a billion-dollar-a-year industry will continue indefinitely at its present scale is uncertain. One good reason for not having national standards of care established by government is to avoid either imposing unsubstantiated treatments or freezing them into current practice.

Scientific and balanced analysis of the costs, risks, and benefits of different treatments is still the exception, not the rule.

4. *"Medical care consists of standard products that can be described precisely and measured meaningfully in standard units such as 'inpatient days,' 'outpatient visits,' or 'doctor office visits.'"*

In fact, medical care is usually anything but a standard product. Much of it is a uniquely personal interaction between two people. The elements of personal trust and confidence are an integral part of the process. Much of the process consists of reassurance and support—*caring* rather than *curing*. What doctors do ranges from the technical marvels of the heart surgeon to marriage counseling by the family doctor, each of which may fill a legitimate human need. A "doctor office visit" might last a few minutes or more than an hour. An "inpatient day" might be accompanied by the use of the most costly and complex technology or be merely a quiet day of rest, with an occasional visit by a nurse.

It is important to correct the misconception that medical care consists of standard products, because it underlies much of the thinking about costs and regulation. People will decry the rapid increase in hospital cost per day without giving recognition to the fact that the services provided during a typical hospital day now are much more complex and use much more elaborate technology than they did a decade ago. Proposals to regulate cost per day or cost per case assume that days or cases are more or less standard, so that the costs of a day in two different hospitals can be compared meaningfully. In fact, before one can make a meaningful comparison, one must specify many conditions, such as severity of illness, the length of stay, and the services provided. The belief that controls on physician fees are a feasible method of controlling the cost of physician services rests on the assumption that "doctor office visits" are more or less standard. They aren't.

Quality of medical care has many different dimensions: accessibility, convenience, style, and effectiveness. There are different systems and styles of care. This variability is desirable. It allows the medical care system to accommodate the preferences and needs of different patients and doctors. But it defies the public-utility regulators, who need standard units, such as passenger miles and kilowatt-hours.

5. *"Much of medical care is a matter of life and death or serious pain or disability."*

This view may come from watching television programs that emphasize the dramatic side of medicine. It is a foundation for the assertion that "health care is a right." As a society, we have agreed that all people should have access to life-saving care without regard to income, race, or social status.

Of course some medical care is life-saving, and its benefits are obvious and clear-cut. But most medical care is not a life-or-death matter at all. Even in the case of care for life-threatening diseases, the effectiveness of much care is measured in terms of small changes in life expectancy (for example, changes in the probability of surviving another year), as opposed to complete cures. Most medical care is a matter of "quality of life." Much of it is concerned with the relief of pain or dysfunction, with caring and reassurance.

All this is not to diminish the importance or value of medical care. But it does suggest that we are dealing with matters of darker or lighter shades of grey, conflicting values, and not clear-cut cases of life or death. Recognizing this makes it much less clear what it is that people have a "right" to or what is "necessary" as opposed to "unnecessary."

6. *"More medical care is better than less care."*

There is a tremendous amount of bias in favor of more care versus less. For example, the observation that physicians in group practices hospitalize their patients much less than do their fellow doctors in traditional solo practice is much more likely to cause suspicion that they are denying their patients necessary care than that the solo-practice doctors are providing too much care.

A. L. Cochrane, a British physician, supplied a nice example of this bias. Dr. H. G. Mather and colleagues in the National Health Service in Bristol did a randomized clinical trial comparing home and hospital treatment of uncomplicated heart attack (acute myocardial infarction) victims.[6] They found that patients cared for in the coronary care units (CCUs) of hospitals survived in no greater proportion than did those cared for at home. Cochrane wrote:

> There is a great deal of bias, and a considerable amount of vested interest. The bias is beautifully illustrated by a story of the early days of Mather's trial. The first report after a few months of the trial showed a slightly greater death-rate in those treated in hospital than those treated at home. Some one reversed the figures and showed them to a CCU enthusiast who immediately declared that the trial was unethical and must be stopped at once. When, however, he was shown the table the correct way round he could not be persuaded to declare CCUs unethical![7]

In fact, more care may not be better than less care. More care may just be useless. Drs. Hill, Hampton, and Mitchell of Nottingham General

Hospital recently repeated Dr. Mather's trial and got a similar result.[8] Of 500 patients whose general practitioners called for the mobile coronary-care unit (a specially equipped ambulance with a doctor), 70 percent were suspected of having a myocardial infarction. Of these, 24 percent were excluded from the trial and were hospitalized because of their medical condition or lack of suitable home environment. The rest were assigned by random method to home or hospital. The result for these patients was no discernable benefit from costly coronary-care units compared with less costly home care. In many cases there may be nothing that medical care can do other than to relieve the patient's discomfort, and this relief may be accomplished as well or better at home as in a costly hospital bed.

Of course, in some cases more care will be better than less. But not in all cases. Above some minimum level that might be provided at a much lower per capita cost, more medical care may yield little, if any, discernible health benefit. This view is supported by two studies of the relationship of health resources to health indicators in different parts of the United States. One study looked at the health status of people living in different places as measured by such things as blood pressure, cholesterol concentration, abnormal electrocardiogram, and abnormal chest X-rays.[9] The other looked at infant mortality and age-adjusted overall mortality.[10] Each attempted to correlate these indicators with such measures of health resources as numbers of doctors and variables such as income, education, and occupation. Both found little or no significant relationship between health resources and health status.

More medical care may actually be harmful. There is such a thing as physician-caused (known as "iatrogenic") disease. People do die or are seriously injured on the operating table, and some are injured or die from the complications of anesthesia. Around 1950 Paul Lembcke, M.D., of Johns Hopkins did a comparative study of death rates from appendicitis (including dying from surgery) in twenty-three different hospital service areas in New York State.[11] He found that the per capita rate of appendectomy in some areas was more than twice that in other areas, even after adjusting for the age and sex composition of the populations. In the absence of evidence to the contrary, Lembcke assumed no differences in the incidence of appendicitis among these rather homogeneous areas. He also found that areas with the highest per capita rates of appendectomy had the highest rates of death from appendicitis. This is the opposite of what one would expect, since appendectomies are done to prevent death from appendicitis. In 1971 two German medical investigators, S. Lichtner and M. Pflanz, reported similar results for Germany.[12] Although the interpretation of these data is being debated, it would appear that some Germans and New Yorkers would have been better off if their appendixes had been left alone!

Philip R. Lee, M.D., former Assistant Secretary of HEW for Health, has determined that excessive medical care may be harmful to your health.

In a study with Milton Silverman, Ph.D., he estimated that "adverse drug reactions," that is, seriously harmful unintended effects of legally available drugs administered in normal doses for the diagnosis, prevention, or treatment of a disease

> occur by the thousands or tens of thousands every day. They kill more victims than does cancer of the breast. They rank among the top ten causes of hospitalization. In the United States alone, they are held accountable for as many as fifty million hospital patient-days a year.[13]

Excessive antibiotics can encourage the development of resistant strains of bacteria. X-rays can cause harm. These and many other examples suggest that a financing system that motivates giving *more* rather than less care is not necessarily leading doctors to give *better* care or to produce better health.

7. *"People have no control over the timing of their need for medical care. Whatever care is needed is needed right away."*

Many people seem to think of the need for medical care as if it were all the result of accidents. Of course, some is. That is one reason why the casualty-insurance model seems to fit.

But a great deal of medical care is elective with respect to timing or is predictable six months or a year in advance. I have not seen a systematic study of this point, but I believe that well over half of all medical care spending is for the treatment of chronic conditions, for care postponable for a year without great risk or suffering, or is elective with respect to timing (for example, a decision to become pregnant or to undergo corrective orthopaedic surgery). How people can use this control to their advantage was illustrated by one California family that had an annual choice between a "low-option" insurance plan with high deductibles and low benefits and membership in a health maintenance organization (HMO), with comprehensive benefits paid in full. The family chose the "low-option" plan in order to pay low premiums, until the discovery that all four children needed open-heart surgery. At the next annual enrollment, the family switched and had the heart surgery at the expense of the HMO. At the subsequent enrollment period, the family switched back to get the low premiums again. Less spectacular examples are commonplace.

The ability of people to control the timing of their need for medical care is another reason why the casualty insurance model fails to fit the facts of medical care. Although the need for some care is acute, the timing of the need for much care is controllable. This puts special requirements on the design of a health insurance system. For example, people cannot be free to buy or not to buy health insurance or to switch from a very limited to a very comprehensive coverage at the time of medical need. For if they were, they could take advantage of the system, go without paying premiums until they expected to need care, and then buy insurance. The system would break down. There would be no "insurance."

WHY FINANCIAL INCENTIVES MAKE A DIFFERENCE

When thinking about medical care, then, we should think in terms of a variety of legitimate treatments for each condition, with their relative merits in a particular case depending on the unique circumstances and values of the people involved. We should remember that there is pervasive uncertainty and that medicine is more an art based on judgment than a science based on calculation. Medical care deals more with the quality of life than with the quantity (length) of life. The "product" does not come in standard units. Medical care is a matter of subtle and complex judgments about more versus less, and more may often not be better. This should make it easier to understand how the institutional arrangements, including economic considerations, can come to play a large role in medical decision making.

If medical diagnoses were always clear-cut, if the best treatment were always obvious, if the element of science were large, if the timing of care were determined by medical necessity, and especially if medical care were mostly a matter of life and death, it would be easier to understand how people could believe that the institutional arrangements for providing medical care, including the financial incentives, would be irrelevant to the amounts and kinds of care provided. This kind of medicine would fit into both the casualty-insurance and public-utility models. Making it free at the time of service would not lead patients to demand more of it. Every medical treatment would be "necessary" or "unnecessary," and medical review boards could audit physician performance if unnecessary care were suspected.

Making the decision to use medical care free or almost free to consumers is bound to lead them to resolve their doubts in favor of more, and more costly, care than if they had to pay for it themselves. And think of the physicians, with their concern for the patient and a humanitarian desire to do everything possible to help alleviate suffering, professional standards that emphasize the most advanced technology, and concern over the threat of malpractice suits in a society that believes that more care is always better than less. If in addition to all that, the financing arrangements make the care free to the patient and also yield more revenue to the doctor for giving more, and more costly, care, it should not be difficult to see how fee-for-service payment contributes to ever more costly care.

Studies show that institutional settings and financial incentives do make a difference in the behavior of patients and doctors. For example, Anne Scitovsky, a leading health services researcher, did a study of visits to the doctor by Stanford University employees and their families cared for under a prepaid plan with the Palo Alto Medical Clinic. [14] In 1966 such visits were fully paid in advance by the monthly premiums. This led to such high use of services and costs that in 1967, the plan was changed to require the families to pay one-quarter of each doctor bill. In 1968 the same people's visits to the doctor's office decreased by 25 percent. (The decline in hospital visits was by only 3 percent.) As far as Mrs. Scitovsky and other investigators could tell, the introduction of this financial disincentive was the only thing that had changed between the two years.

Incentives for the physicians can also be important; indeed, they are much more important than patient incentives from an economic point of view, because physicians make the costly decisions. George Monsma, Jr., an economist at Amherst College, highlighted this by comparing the number of operations per capita in groups of employees and their families, some of whom were cared for under group-practice prepayment plans, and some of whom were cared for under traditional insured fee-for-service plans.[15] In the group-practice prepayment plans the surgery is free to the beneficiary, and the doctors get no more money for doing the surgery, because they are paid on the basis of a monthly per capita payment that is independent of the number of services performed. Under the traditional insured fee-for-service plans, the beneficiary pays 20 to 25 percent of the doctor bill, and the doctor gets more money for doing the operation than for not doing it.

The consumer incentive would be to have less surgery under the insured plan. But Monsma found significantly higher rates of surgery under the insured plan, thus lending support to the view that the physicians' incentives (which are in turn a function of how the physicians are organized and paid) dominate decision making on use of surgery. Numerous other comparative studies have reached similar conclusions.[16]

To observe that financial incentives play an important role in the use of medical services is not to imply that they are the only, or even the most important, factor. Physicians are concerned primarily with curing their sick patients, regardless of the cost. That ethic has been instilled in them through years of arduous training. Many take a failure to cure a sick patient as a personal defeat. When we are sick, we want our doctors to be concerned with curing us and nothing else. Physicians and other health professionals are also motivated by a desire to achieve professional excellence and the esteem of their peers and the public. But their use of resources is inevitably shaped by financial incentives. Physicians who survive and prosper must ultimately do what brings in money and curtail those activities that lose money.

WHY THE CASUALTY INSURANCE MODEL DOESN'T FIT MEDICAL CARE WELL

All this should not be surprising until we reflect that we have imposed on medical care a financial system, borrowed from casualty insurance, that assumes that financial incentives do not play an important part in decisions about the use of services.

Think about casualty insurance. The hurricane did or did not damage your house. You did or did not have a collision. Few people will choose to drive carelessly merely because they have insurance. If you have an insured loss, you report it to the insurance company. A claims adjustor negotiates with you a fixed value for the loss. It is not open-ended. It is a reasonable working assumption that the existence of insurance will not have a major impact on the amount of the losses. Of course, the assumption does not fit perfectly. People who have insurance are likely to demand more and better repairs than those who do not. And commercial arson (deliberately setting fire to a property in order to collect the insurance) is a significant problem for fire insurers. But these departures from the assumption can be rendered manageable by the use of inspectors, claims adjustors, and coinsurance.

As I observed at the beginning of the chapter, most people think of the need for medical care in similar terms. You are unambiguously either sick or well. If you are sick, you go to the doctor, who diagnoses your illness, applies the standard treatment, and sends a bill for the "usual, customary, and reasonable" fee, all or most of which is paid by your insurance company. The insurer assumes that the fee is set in a normal economic marketplace.

But the model does not fit the facts of medical care at all well. For example, the doctor's position is very different from that of the insurance claims adjustor. In most cases the doctor cannot set a fixed price for a cure in advance. There is too much uncertainty. And his or her responsibility is to cure the patient, not to limit the cost to a fixed amount. The fact that most people are insured means that they have little or no financial incentive to question the value of or need for services. It also means that the physician and the hospital management can feel quite free to offer the most costly care, whether or not it does the patient any more good than less costly care, without the concern that the cost will burden their individual patients. Uncertainties are usually resolved in favor of the more costly alternative.

These insights also help explain why qualitative distinctions such as one finds in legal usage are not very helpful. One simply cannot divide all medical care into the categories "necessary" and "unnecessary." What is "necessary" care? Is "necessary" care limited to treatment of serious pain or life-threatening conditions? If it were, a great deal of care would not be "necessary." Even in life-and-death cases, the concept of "necessary" poorly describes many situations. Suppose that a patient with terminal cancer has 99-to-1 odds of dying within a year. Suppose that treatment costing $20,000 will reduce those odds to 97 to 1. Would that be "necessary" or "unnecessary" care? There are doubtless examples that most observers would judge to be "unnecessary." But the fact that two doctors disagree and that the doctor offering the "second opinion" says that the operation is "unnecessary" does not make it so.

Similarly, forceful assertions that "health care is a right" do not help in this large grey zone. In view of the variety of systems and styles of care and treatments, exactly what is a *right*? A *right* to *anything* health care providers can do to make you feel better? That interpretation would make "health care is a right" mean "money is no object." Our society cannot afford and will not support such a generous definition.

The concepts and language most useful for analyzing the problem of health care costs are concepts that have been developed for decision making under uncertainty and for choices of "a little more or a little less." We need to think in terms of judgments about probabilites and in terms of the balancing of various costs, risks, and benefits. The issues are not, for example, "complete care vs. no care for a heart-attack patient." Rather, they are more of the character "seven vs. fourteen or twenty-one days in the hospital after a heart attack." What is the medical value of the extra days? How do they affect the probability that the patient will be alive a year later? What do they cost, not only in resources measured in money, but also in other terms? Are the extra benefits worth the extra costs? These are the kinds of questions we must keep asking if we want to make sense out of the problem and to get good value for the money we spend on health care. They are matters of judgment, possibly aided by calculation.

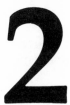

Irrational Incentives and the Growth of Health Care Spending

THE GROWTH OF HEALTH CARE SPENDING AND THE CHANGING PATTERN OF FINANCE

Growth of Spending

National health care spending reached $192 billion in 1978, about four and one-half times its 1965 level.[1] The year 1965 is a useful base for comparison because Medicare and Medicaid were enacted then and became effective in 1966. In 1965 national health care spending was 6.2 percent of the gross national product; in 1978, 9.1 percent. The composition of this spending is shown in Table 1. Physicians' services account for

TABLE 1   National Health Expenditures, 1965 and 1978 ($billions)

	1965	1978	Percent of 1978 Total	Average Annual Growth
Hospital Care	$13.9	$ 76.0	40%	14.0%
Physicians' Services	8.5	35.3	18	11.6
Dentists' Services	2.8	13.3	7	12.7
Drugs and Drug Sundries	5.8	15.1	8	7.6
Nursing-home Care	2.1	15.8	8	16.8
All Other	9.9	36.9	19	—
Total	**$43.0**	**$192.4**	**100**	**12.2**

Source: Robert M. Gibson, "National Health Expenditures, 1978," Health Care Financing Review 1 (Summer 1979): 1–36.

about 18 percent of the total and have grown at a rate slightly less than the total. The largest single component is hospital care, which was about 40 percent of the total. With the exception of nursing home care, hospital care was also the fastest-growing component. Thus government cost-containment efforts have focused on it.

About half of the increase in spending can be attributed to general inflation in the economy. In addition, the United States population in 1978 was about 12 percent greater than in 1965. So a more meaningful comparison would be between real (that is, adjusted for general inflation) per capita spending, as is shown in Table 2. Although real per capita spending in total doubled between 1965 and 1978, spending for hospital care increased 2.5 times and for nursing home care increased 3.4 times.

Changing Sources of Funds

The sources of funds to pay for health services changed markedly over these years. A comparison of 1965 and 1978 is shown in Table 3. Direct payments by patients and their families fell from 53 percent of the total cost of personal health care services to 33 percent. This decrease was made up largely by the federal government, whose contribution went up from 10 percent to 28 percent. Of the grand total of health care spending, including research and administration not included in personal health care services, the contribution of government went up from 25 percent to 41 percent.

What is more significant, from the point of view of financial incentives, is that over these years, the percentage of hospital care paid for by "third parties" (other than by patients directly) went up from 82 percent to 90 percent. The percentage of physicians' services paid by third parties went up from 39 percent of the total to 66 percent. Moreover, most health insurance is written in such a way that once patients have entered the hospital and thereby incurred expenses in excess of the deductibles in

---

TABLE 2   Real Per Capita Health Expenditures, 1965 and 1978 (in 1978 dollars)

	1965	1978	1978 ÷ 1965
Hospital Care	$138	$341	2.5
Physicians' Services	84	158	1.9
Dentists' Services	28	60	2.1
Drugs and Drug Sundries	57	68	1.2
Nursing Home Care	21	71	3.4
All Other	98	165	1.7
Total	**$426**	**$863**	**2.0**

Source: Robert M. Gibson, "National Health Expenditures, 1978," Health Care Financing Review 1 (Summer 1979): 1–36.

TABLE 3   Sources of Personal Health Care Spending, 1965 and 1978

	1965	*1978*
Direct Payments	53%	33%
Private Third-Party Payments	25	28
Federal Government	10	28
State and Local Government	11	11

Source: Robert M. Gibson, "National Health Expenditures, 1978," Health Care Financing Review **1** *(Summer 1979): 1–36.*

their policies, practically 100 percent of any additional cost is paid by public or private insurance.

What Is the Problem?

These data show that there has been a big increase in spending on health care. They do not, in themselves, show that we are spending too much. There is no reason to believe that any particular percentage of the gross national product spent on health care is, of itself, too much or too little. The "right" amount depends on how much people want to spend on health care.

Moreover, there are good and acceptable reasons for much of the increase. Growth in public and private insurance coverage made it possible for many people to obtain care who previously could not afford it, especially the aged and the poor. Advances in technology increased the power of medicine to enhance the quality of life. There are many things that medicine can do today to relieve suffering and restore function that couldn't be done twenty years ago, e.g., hip replacements or restoration of severed limbs. The population has grown older. The health care system took on new assignments, such as in mental health and alcohol and drug abuse. What we now call "the disease of alcoholism," and treat medically, we used to call "drunkenness," and treat in the criminal-justice system. The pay of health care workers was brought up to the level in other industries.[2] Rising incomes and expectations increased consumer demand for health care services. Our present concern with the growth in spending should not mislead us into thinking that it is all bad. Much of it is good.

However, I believe that the growth in health care spending is a serious problem for our society for several reasons. First, public-sector spending on health care increased from $11 billion in 1965 to $78 billion in 1978. Our commitment, as a society, to pay for the care of those who cannot afford adequate care, mainly the aged and the poor, is turning out to cost much more than we expected. It is straining public finances at a time when there are other urgent demands on the federal budget, such as for national defense and tax reduction. Because the growth in productivity in our economy has slowed markedly in recent years, we need, if anything, to reduce taxes in order to reduce the burden on the productive sectors of our economy. There are growing signs of taxpayer resentment and resistance. And we need to reduce the heavy burden of health care costs on American industry in order to free resources for such urgent priorities as energy conversion and development and productivity improvement.

Second, as will be explained in more detail later in this chapter, our present system of health care finance is dominated by irrational cost-increasing incentives. I believe that there is a great deal of waste and a great deal of use of services that yield no discernible benefit in terms of health. My evidence for this is summarized in Chapter 3. I would estimate that with appropriate organization and incentives, we could obtain all of the health benefits our present system provides for a cost that is at least 25 percent less than we will be paying in the absence of reform. This estimate is based on the experiences of organized systems of care that use resources wisely, of the kinds discussed in Chapter 4. Considering the size of our present outlays, now well in excess of $200 billion per year, that is a possibility that must be taken seriously.

MAIN CAUSES OF SPENDING INCREASE

No Rewards for Economy

The main cause of the unjustified and unnecessary increase in costs is the complex of irrational economic incentives inherent in the system of fee-for-service payment for doctors, cost reimbursement for hospitals, and what are called "third-party payors." (A rational economic incentive is one that rewards providers of care for giving better care at less cost.)

Fee for service rewards the doctor with more revenue for providing more, and more costly, services, whether or not more is truly beneficial to the patient. Cost reimbursement rewards the hospital with more revenue for generating more costs. And because most fees, costs, and charges are paid by third-party payors (mainly Blue Cross–Blue Shield, commercial insurance companies, Medicare, and Medicaid), most consumers are insulated from concern about costs and have, at most, a weak financial incentive to question the need for or value of services. Nor is there an incentive to seek out a less costly provider or style of care.

The economic factors are important, but the important factors are not all economic. The financial incentives are reinforced by the demands and expectations of anxious patients, "defensive medicine" as a response to the fear of malpractice suits, and the prestige associated with costly technological care. There are many rewards for cost-increasing behavior and virtually no rewards for economy. Such a system must produce inflation in prices and waste in the use of resources.

I like to describe this financing system as being like an "expensive lunch club." Imagine that you and nineteen friends belong to a lunch club. You agree that you will each pay 5 percent of the total lunch bill for the group. Each member is free to choose whatever he or she wants. Consider the incentives. Suppose you go to lunch one day, feeling that a $2 salad would satisfy your desires and be just fine for your health. You watch your friends order. One orders filet mignon; another, lobster. You calculate that if you order the $12 filet instead of the $2 salad, it will cost you only $.50 more. There is little economic incentive for you to choose the less costly meal. If the waiter expects a tip equal to 10 or 15 percent of the bill, imagine which dishes he will recommend. And if everybody in town is a member of this or a similar club, there is not much incentive for anybody to open an economical restaurant that specializes in healthy $2 salads!

Growth and Impact of Insurance Coverage

In 1962 roughly 130 million Americans, or 70 percent of the civilian population, had private insurance for hospital expenses.[3] In addition, federal, state, and local governments were spending roughly $5 billion per year on personal health care services for the poor, veterans, Defense Department beneficiaries, and others.

Between 1962 and 1972, the number of people covered by private insurance increased by some 25 to 35 million. In 1965 Congress enacted Title XVIII of the Social Security Act—Health Insurance for the Aged, or Medicare—and Title XIX—Grants to States for Medical Assistance Programs, or Medicaid. The Congressional Budget Office estimated in 1976 that about 23 million people were covered by Medicare, about 22 million by Medicaid. Of course, not all of these were net additions to the rolls of the insured, because many of the aged had private insurance before Medicare, and there were federal grants for state programs of medical assistance to the needy before Medicaid. Moreover, coverage of military dependents was expanded in 1966 to cover retirees and their dependents and to dependents of deceased service members. By 1975 the Defense Department covered nearly 7 million people other than active-duty military. In the most thorough study of the subject to date, the Congressional Budget Office estimated that by 1976, some 92 to 95 percent of the population had some health insurance coverage.[4]

Like most aggregate data in the health care field, these data are uncertain and are subject to change. It is very difficult to estimate accurately the percentage of the population that has health insurance. One might think that it would be easy: Just ask each insurer how many people it covers. The main problem with such an approach is that there is a great deal of duplicate coverage. For example, both spouses may work and each cover the family through their respective employers. Estimates of the number of people with duplicate private coverage in 1975 ranged from 34 to 44 million. Some people who are eligible for public insurance also have private coverage. About 17 million of the 23 million people aged sixty-five and over in 1975 carried private insurance in addition to Medicare. The other approach to estimating coverage is to interview households and ask them about their health insurance. The main problem with it is that many people appear to be unaware of their coverage or unwilling to reveal their eligibility for programs for the poor.

In some cases the meaning of the word "covered" or "eligible for coverage" is unclear. For example, the eligibility criteria for Medicaid vary from state to state. In general, the eligible are those in certain categories, such as aged, disabled, and families with dependent children, with incomes below the state-determined eligibility level. But families in the eligible categories with incomes above the eligibility limit become eligible when their incomes, net of medical expenses, fall below the limit. So in a sense a family with an income $10 per month above the eligibility limit has comprehensive coverage with a $10 per month deductible. Is it "covered" by Medicaid?

The economic effect of health insurance is, of course, to reduce the cost of covered services to the insured consumer. Instead of paying the full cost to the economy of a service, the insured consumer pays some fraction of that cost, possibly even zero. Thus any economic restraint on the would-be patient, and any restraint on his or her doctor that comes from knowing that the patient will have to pay the cost of care, is greatly attenuated or even eliminated when the patient is insured.

The data in Table 4, from Harvard University economists Martin Feldstein and Amy Taylor, illustrate this point.[5] Although average hospital cost per patient day increased from $15.62 in 1950 to $151.53 in 1975, the net cost to the consumer in constant 1967 dollars remained virtually unchanged, at about $11.

The large increase in cost of services with no increase in cost to the consumer when he receives the services has, of course, meant large increases in insurance premiums. The question naturally arises, then, of why the increase in premiums has not produced more consumer resistance and, perhaps, decisions to buy less costly insurance covering less costly

---

TABLE 4 Insurance and the Net Cost of Hospital Care

	1950	1975
Average Cost per Patient Day in Current Dollars	$15.62	$151.53
Average Cost per Patient Day in 1967 Dollars	21.66	94.00
Percent Paid by Consumers, Net of Public and Private Insurance	49.6%	11.9%
Net Cost per Patient Day in 1967 Dollars	$10.75	$11.19

Source: Martin S. Feldstein and Amy Taylor, The Rapid Rise of Hospital Costs, *staff report, Washington, D.C.: Council on Wage and Price Stability, January 1977.*

benefits. The answer is that most people have their premiums paid, in large part or in total, by employer or government and have no choice in the matter. In 1974 the benefits of 68 percent of the workers in those private-industry health plans covering more than twenty-five workers were paid for entirely by the employer. Similarly, the hospital-insurance part of Medicare is paid for largely by payroll taxes; the physician-service part, heavily subsidized by general tax revenues. Medicaid benefits are fully paid by federal and state governments. So most people are quite unaware of the costs of their health insurance.

Impact of the Tax Laws

The tax laws exclude employer contributions to the health insurance (or health care) of employees and dependents from the employee's taxable income subject to federal and state income taxes. Employer health-benefit contributions are also excluded from the pay on which employer and employee social security taxes are based. That is, if your employer contributes $1200 to your health insurance premiums, that amount is tax-free pay. If, instead, the employer pays you $1200 in cash and tells you to go out and buy your own insurance, you and the employer must first pay a total of roughly $300 to $600 in federal and state income taxes and social security taxes on the $1200. (The exact amount will depend on your tax bracket. Some will be lower than 30 percent or higher than 50 percent.) Thus there is a large financial advantage to the employee's getting health insurance through an employer instead of purchasing it on his or her own. In 1979 this favorable tax treatment of health benefits meant that the federal and state governments received about $14 billion less in tax revenues than they would have otherwise.[6]

The incentives created by this tax treatment have had profound consequences for the development of health insurance. First, the tax laws have put health benefits under the control of employers and, where there are unions, under the joint control of labor and management. On the positive side, employers and unions can act as informed buyers for employees, and the employee group or union membership serves as a logical basis for economic group purchase. But there are also negative aspects. Employers and unions have their own goals. Employers use health benefits as a tool for attracting qualified employees or as a way of discouraging unionization. Union leaders see health benefits as a prize to be won at the bargaining table and as a way of making the union appear to be the worker's benefactor. The implicit message is: "You have better health benefits because you are a member of this union, and we are its leaders; stay with us, and next year, we'll get you free glasses and dental care." Health benefits thus take on a political significance beyond their purely economic value. The specific shape of the health-benefits package becomes a by-product of the collective-bargaining process and not necessarily the best use of the health dollars. All this puts the emphasis on benefits specific to the particular employer or union rather than on better or more economical health care for the community as a whole. And it creates a continual pressure for more extensive benefits.

Second, the tax laws motivate employees to take more of their gross compensation in health benefits than they would if employer contributions were taxed like any other income. If employees take an additional dollar of gross compensation in wages or salary, they get to keep roughly $0.50 to $0.70 after taxes. If they take it in health benefits, they get the full dollar. Thus the cost to the employee, in foregone after-tax income, of an extra dollar of health benefits is $0.50 to $0.70. This is becoming more important as inflation and increasing payroll taxes push us all into higher tax brackets.

Consider a hypothetical employee whose total compensation has been fixed by agreement with her employer. Assume that she has a choice between two health plans, one costing $1000 and the other $1200 a year. Assume that she is in the 40 percent combined tax bracket (that is, of each additional $100 of gross pay her employer pays, income and social security taxes take $40.) Assume further that the employer will pay the whole premium of either plan and $200 more in salary if she selects the less costly health plan. (One important problem, discussed in Chapter 5, is that most employers don't offer such a choice.) By taking the $1200 plan, the employee's salary is $200 less than it would otherwise be, but her take-home pay is only $120 less. Thus in effect the government is paying $80, or 40 percent of the extra cost of the more expensive plan. In this way the tax laws subsidize the choice of more costly health plans. Because of the tax laws, it is attractive for employees to have the employer pay even for routine costs that could easily be budgeted by the employee, such as for eye glasses and routine dentistry. Employees have incentives to purchase more health care benefits with their employers' before-tax dollars than they would purchase with their own after-tax dollars.

Third, the tax laws make it logical for the employer to pay 100 percent of the premium for all of the health insurance the employee wants to buy. That is, if the employer and the worker have agreed on a total sum for compensation, including health benefits, the employee will pay less taxes if the employer pays the whole insurance premium and pays the rest to the employee as wages. One effect of the growing pattern of 100 percent employer-paid benefits has been to make employees uninformed about and insensitive to the costs of health insurance.

In Chapter 5 I will explain why it would be desirable for every employer to offer his employees several health plans from which to choose and to contribute in the form of a fixed dollar amount. Let me note here that the practice of the great majority of employers has been to offer a *single* health insurance plan. Thus in the manner in which it has been exercised, employer control has served to create a barrier to health plan competition.

If one plan is to be offered, almost inevitably it will be a "free choice of doctor" plan. Employers and unions are understandably reluctant to attempt to restrict employee choices of doctor. "Company store medicine" is not popular in the United States. The effect is that the employee can elect the most costly doctor at no economic penalty. Employers who offer such insurance are, in effect, saying to the most costly providers that their costs will be paid, almost no matter what they are. (I use the term "most costly providers" to refer to those who generate the most total costs per person cared for or per case and not necessarily for those who charge the highest prices. A high-priced doctor might not be among the most costly if he or she orders fewer tests or less hospitalization.) The situation resembles "the expensive lunch club," described earlier.

In Chapter 7 I will explain how the link between jobs and health insurance creates complexity and leads to gaps in coverage. Let me note here simply that the tax laws are an important reason for the existence of this link.

Fee for Service

Most doctors in the United States are paid on the basis of "fee for service," essentially a piece-work basis, rather than some other arrangement, such as a monthly retainer fee for providing comprehensive care or an all-inclusive charge per case. In the fee-for-service system, doctors charge separately for each service performed. If they do more services, they charge more. This, of course, gives them an incentive to do more, even if more yields a negligible benefit to the patient. Typically, the doctor is both the advisor to the patient on the need for services and the provider to the patient of physician services. (The doctor may also advise and provide lab tests, X-rays, injections, and other services.) The conflict of interest should be apparent. As the element of uncertainty in medical practice is quite large, the physician has wide latitude to recommend more services that might do some good. And, of course, the insured patient has little or no financial incentive to question the need for more services. In prescribing more for an insured patient, the doctor can usually feel that he or she is acting in the patient's best interest. It is the combination of insured patients and fee-for-service doctors that is an especially potent force for increased spending.

The incentives in the fee-for-service system also reward more costly types of care rather than less costly care. Doctors are paid more per hour for doing new technologic procedures than for such services as examining and advising patients. Mark Blumberg, M.D., a health care analyst with Kaiser Foundation Health Plan, observed that "when technological improvements occur, the original high price is maintained even though production costs fall. . . . This is probably the main reason for the high profitability of diagnostic X-rays, electrocardiographs, blood chemistry tests and even injections."[7]

Alvin Thompson, M.D., gave the following example in his September 1978 valedictory address as President of the Washington State Medical Society:

> We must think about the effect of financial incentives on what we do. I am a gastroenterologist and an endoscopist. Suppose a patient comes in complaining of diarrhea. If I do a colonoscopy examination, many third party payers will readily pay nearly $400. That is ten times the forty dollars I might receive if I just talked with the patient for an hour to find out what he was doing that was causing the diarrhea. Yet, from the point of view of his health, listening might be a better way for me to spend the hour. We must ask ourselves whether such incentives are leading us to do more costly procedures than would be best for our patients.

Dr. Blumberg also found that the structure of fees provides strong financial incentives to care for patients in the hospital rather than in the office. The key point of his analysis is summarized in Table 5. In 1974 an internist saw an average of 2.47 patients per hour when caring for patients in the office, 3.69 per hour, or 49 percent more, when seeing patients on hospital rounds. Yet the fee for a follow-up visit in the hospital was 34 percent higher than for a follow-up visit in the office. The net result was that the doctor's revenue per hour when working in the hospital was twice that realized when working in the office. The differential in net revenue is even greater because the physician does not need to use as much office staff and overhead for a hospital visit.

Fee for service is advantageous for doctors. It gives them maximum control over their incomes and wide latitude to set their own fees. Very few patients would think to negotiate with their doctors over fees, especially when they are sick and in need of the doctor's help and goodwill, which is the only time the subject is likely to arise. Even more important, fees are not good material for economic comparison. They don't tell you much about the total cost for a cure, which is what you would want to

---

TABLE 5   Revenue per Hour for Hospital and Office Visits, 1974

| Specialty | Patient Visits Per Hour | | Relative Fee Follow-up Visits Hospital ÷ Office Visit | Relative Revenue Per Hour, Hospital ÷ Office |
	Office	Hospital Rounds		
General Practice	3.87	3.08	1.46	1.16
Internal Medicine	2.47	3.69	1.34	2.00
Surgery	3.19	4.33	1.48	2.01
Obstetrics-Gynecology	3.36	3.99	1.30	1.54
Pediatrics	3.44	3.82	1.34	1.49

Source: Mark S. Blumberg, "Rational Provider Prices: Provider Price Changes for Improved Health Care Use," Health Handbook, ed. George K. Chacko, Amsterdam: North Holland Publishing, 1979. Used with permission.

know if you were cost-conscious. The well-insured patient has little reason to question fees or the need for services. Thus insurance with "free choice of doctor" effectively rules out economic competition among doctors. Fee for service is also most compatible with the individual entrepreneurial practice style and professional independence traditionally preferred by most physicians. Any other mode of payment is likely to involve more people and to reduce the physician's independence.

However, fee for service is not advantageous for consumers. A sensible buyer of physician services might well prefer to negotiate an annual retainer fee for which a group of doctors would agree in advance to provide all care if and when it proves necessary. Such a retainer, or per capita payment, could be negotiated when the buyer is well and able to consider the retainer fees of several physician groups. However, the development of such arrangements has been actively discouraged by the medical profession.[8]

The Key Role of the Physician

As we have seen, although their gross incomes account for only about 18 percent of total health care spending, physicians control or influence most of the rest. By one estimate, physicians directly control 70 percent of all personal health care expenditures.[9] Even though it may not appear so on an organization chart, physicians are the primary decision makers in the health care system. But the present structure of the system assigns very little responsibility to them for the economic consequences of their decisions. Most doctors have no idea what hospital costs, pharmacy costs, and other ancillary patient-care costs actually are.[10] As recently as 1979, hospital efforts to educate physicians about the costs of the things they order were being treated as major news items. The system gives physicians little or no incentive to find out about cost or to act on the information if they have it. Their professional values combine with the financial incentives and other factors to minimize concern over cost and to foster cost-increasing behavior. If the decision makers in a system are not concerned with cost-effectiveness, the system will not be cost-effective.

But the physicians' impact on hospital costs cannot be characterized merely as one of neutrality based on ignorance. Paul Ellwood, M.D., President of InterStudy, put it this way: "Hospitals don't have patients. Hospitals have doctors, and doctors have patients. Therefore, hospitals compete for doctors." And they compete in costly ways such as providing house staff (resident physicians) to do much of the work and to eliminate the inconvenience of night or weekend visits. Hospitals also compete for doctors by offering them the use of the latest and most complex equipment, the use of convenient offices at subsidized rental rates, and even guarantees of a certain income.[11] All of these costs are passed on to the third-party payors.

Cost Reimbursement for Hospitals

Most hospitals today are paid on the basis of either costs or charges. Medicare, Medicaid, and most Blue Cross plans pay on the basis of *cost*. Each of these payors has its own regulations governing what it considers "allowable costs" and may not pay 100 percent of costs as seen by the hospital. The essential point is that if the hospital's "allowable costs" for caring for the beneficiaries of these payors go up by $1, its reimbursement will go up by $1, so there is no financial incentive to hold costs down. Medicare has criteria governing what it considers a "reasonable" routine cost per patient day. ("Routine cost" refers to room and board or "hotel" costs plus routine nursing. It does not include lab tests, surgery, and other specialized services.) But these have not proved to be effective cost controls, because the "reasonableness" of a hospital's costs is judged in relation to the costs of other hospitals. The controls penalize the most costly hospitals, but do not effectively restrain increases in the costs of the majority of hospitals that are not far from the median. Moreover, "routine costs" per day can be reduced in ways that increase total costs. For example, hospitals may perform more ancillary services or encourage longer inpatient stays, so that overheads may be spread over more units of service.

Most private insurers, some Blue Cross plans, and uninsured private paying patients pay "charges," that is, the prices set by the hospital. Some insurance policies pay an "indemnity," a flat amount per service, and the patient pays the excess, if any. Such policies are often combined with "major medical" insurance that pays 80 percent of the excess after a deductible is satisfied. There is little economic restraint on charges, because practically all patients have insurance. The only restraint on hospital administrators' setting charges is to avoid being "unreasonable." "Reasonableness" is usually judged in relation to the costs and the charges of other hospitals.

This system actually punishes some important kinds of economical behavior. Suppose that a hospital administrator sincerely believed that many people in her community would be better off with a less costly style of care. Suppose she were able to do such things as institute tighter controls on use of surgery and laboratory and avoid buying certain costly diagnostic equipment by referring patients to other hospitals. The first thing she would experience would be a loss in revenue. For each dollar she cut from cost, she would lose about a dollar in reimbursement. The next thing she would experience is a loss in physician staff as doctors took their patients to the hospitals offering better equipment and looser controls. So she would be punished for her efforts. And, assuming that the hospital insurance premiums of the people in the community reflect the average costs of patients over an area much wider than the hospital's service area, there would be no way that she could return much of the savings to the citizens in her community. There would not be many grateful citizens at her going-away dinner.

The Passive Role of Third-Party Payors

In the jargon of health care, there are consumers (patients), providers of care (mainly doctors and hospitals), and "third parties" (the bill payors). Usually the terms "third-party payor" or "intermediary" are used interchangeably with "insurer." But not all the third-party payors are insurance companies. The list also includes the federal government, state governments, and employers, some of whom pay their employees' health care bills directly, with or without claims-review services provided by insurance companies.

A key fact about the third parties is that they receive the bill after the costs have been incurred. They are not involved before the fact in the planning, organization, and delivery of services. All they can do is to decide whether or not to pay the bill. But this would be a formidable task if they attempted a serious review of each bill. All told, Americans made more than a billion visits to their doctors in 1976, had about 278 million days of care in short-term hospital stays, made 190 million outpatient visits to community hospitals, not to mention the almost uncountable number of laboratory tests, prescriptions, and other health care–related goods and services. In fact, for the most part, all the third parties can do is to "manage by exception," that is, look for the unusual, for the cases that lie outside statistical norms. Of necessity, the "normal care" goes unreviewed.

Upon receiving a bill, a third-party payor basically has three alternatives. (1) It can pay the bill. (2) It can object to the bill as unusual or unreasonable or not related to costs, in which case it tries to make the provider absorb the bill or at least the excess amount. This action may have some deterrent effect on providers and thus contribute to cost control. But it cannot influence the great bulk of the costs, because it is focused on exceptional cases. Most insurers make such objections in only a small percentage of cases. (3) It can reject the claim on the grounds that it is not a covered benefit. The effect is to shift the cost to the beneficiary.

Private insurers usually do not have a strong incentive to control costs, because of the way they set their premiums. Most premiums, at least for large employee groups, are set on the basis of what is called "experience rating." This means that the premium is set equal to the actual health care costs experienced by the insured group, plus an additional amount for administrative cost and profit. In some cases the premium is set in advance. If it turns out not to have been enough to cover costs, the insurer may include the overrun in the next year's premium. In some cases the premium is adjusted at the end of the year to reflect the actual costs that were incurred. Recognizing that the costs are actually being paid with their money and not the insurers', many employers are now switching to what is called "administrative services only" (ASO) contracts with insurance companies. The insurance company then merely processes the claims and pays them with a check drawn on the employer's bank account. In either case the insurer is working with the employer's money and is not strongly motivated to control health care costs.

Moreover, both insurers and employers are reluctant to take any actions that would upset employees. This might occur if either refused to pay a bill or antagonized a patient's doctor. Such action might appear to be an attempt to evade a contractual obligation. The potential savings in any individual case are likely to appear small compared with the potential cost of contesting a claim submitted by either an employee or physician.

The government as insurer has more of an incentive to control costs, because the health care costs it pays are a budgetary item. More money spent for medical care means either less for other programs or higher deficits or taxes. The Medicare program has developed an extremely complex system for determining allowable costs and fees. In the case of hospitals, Medicare has a "screen" for determining reasonableness of routine hospital costs per day. In the case of physician fees, Medicare has developed a "screen" for what is "reasonable," based on charges that are "customary and prevailing." The limits were set based on fees in 1971, updated each year by an overall economic index of general earnings levels and physicians' expenses. The index grows less rapidly than physician fees in general. The result is that the percentage of claims in which physicians would accept the Medicare-determined fee as full payment dropped from about 62 percent of all Medicare claims in 1969 to 52 percent in 1975. When the doctor does not accept the Medicare fee as payment in full, the patient has to pay the difference. Thus Medicare is not controlling these costs, but is merely shifting them to the beneficiaries. After a deductible has been satisfied by the patient, Medicare pays 80 percent of "reasonable" fee. In many cases this turns out to be more like 50 percent of the actual fee.

The third parties have proved to be weak, indeed powerless, to control costs, and this is largely for a simple reason. The real power to control costs is the power to refuse to buy if the price is not right. But neither third-party payors nor employers have that power as long as the beneficiary has the right of "free choice of doctor." As long as we preserve the right of "free choice of doctor," only the beneficiary has the power to refuse to buy from the more costly provider. But the beneficiary has no incentive to seek out less costly providers, for the insurance premium is the same whether he chooses the more or the less costly providers. (As one member of a large group, the extra costs a beneficiary generates by choosing a more costly provider are spread thinly over all the members, so one's choice has a negligible effect on one's own premium. Recall the "expensive lunch club" analogy.)

It would seem reasonable, as an alternative, to let the beneficiary choose among several groups of providers, with different insurance premiums for each reflecting the cost-generating experience of each. The beneficiary could then bear the extra costs or realize the savings associated with his or her choice.

More Doctors

There was a time when economists and others believed that the cause of high and rising physician fees was monopolistic restriction of entry into the medical profession. In a 1976 suit against the American Medical Association, the Federal Trade Commission included that charge. The policy prescription seemed clear: Increase the supply of physicians in order to drive down the price of physicians' services and the costs of medical care. This prescription ignored some of the unusual characteristics of the market for physicians' services, especially the impact of widespread insurance.

So starting in the early 1960s, the capacity of American medical schools was expanded from about 8300 entering students in 1960 to 14,200 by 1973. For a time, the immigration laws were also changed to favor the entry of "foreign medical graduates." The number of active physicians per 100,000 population increased from 140 in 1960 to 174 by 1975 and has been projected by the Department of Health, Education, and Welfare to reach 242 by 1990. This increase has had no apparent depressing effect on health care costs or even physician fees. What happened?

In 1972 Victor Fuchs and Marcia Kramer, then with the National Bureau of Economic Research, published a detailed study, *Determinants of Expenditures for Physicians Services in the United States 1948–1968*. They concluded:

> The demand for physicians' services appears to be significantly influenced by the number of physicians available. . . . Physician supply, across states is positively related to price. . . . Because physicians can and do determine the demand for their own services to a considerable extent, we should be wary of plans which assume that the cost of medical care would be reduced by increasing the supply of physicians.[12]

In other words, more doctors per capita means more doctoring and higher prices, not the lower prices that are supposed to follow an increase in supply.

The hypothesis that doctors create demand for their services touched off a lively debate among economists.[13] Critics argued that the finding defied the laws of supply and demand, that the Fuchs-Kramer theory failed to explain what did determine fees if supply and demand didn't, and that studies using other data did not clearly show this phenomenon. In 1978 Victor Fuchs published another study focused on the supply of surgeons and the demand for surgical operations. Again, he found that other things equal, a 10 percent increase in the surgeon/population ratio results in about a 3 percent increase in per capita utilization. Moreover, differences in supply seem to have a perverse effect on fees, raising them when the surgeon/population ratio increases.[14]

However the issue of doctor-created demand is eventually resolved, this conclusion does seem to emerge quite clearly: Physicians practicing in areas where there are more doctors per capita charge more, see fewer patients, work fewer hours, and make roughly the same net incomes as do those practicing in areas with fewer doctors per capita. Princeton economist Uwe Reinhardt made the point with an interregional comparison, summarized in Table 6.[15] Thus more doctors per capita will mean more cost per capita.

Economists have not agreed on an explanation of this unusual economic behavior. Clearly, the existence of widespread insurance is one key factor. One explanation that has been offered is the "target income hypothesis." As the number of doctors increases and the workload per doctor falls, doctors need to charge more to make the incomes to which they feel entitled.

Technology

Another factor associated with increased spending has been the tremendous growth, during the 1960s and 1970s, in the power, complexity, and cost of medical technology. To give a few examples is to risk overstating the significance of the large-scale "spectaculars" and thereby understating the significance of the widespread application of all kinds of new technologies throughout medical practice. Still, a brief review of a few examples will help us to appreciate that the bundle of services bought

---

TABLE 6   Regional Differences in Certain Health Care Statistics, United States 1969–1970

	New England States	East–South Central States
Active MDs in patient care per 100,000 population	161	95
Average fee for routine follow-up office visit		
Internal Medicine	$9.40	$7.70
General Surgery	9.76	6.85
Annual patient visits per MD	4,808	8,408
Average number of hours worked in patient care		
per MD	2,128	2,303
Average net income (all specialties)	$38,019	$41,963

Source: Uwe E. Reinhardt, Physician Productivity and the Demand for Health Manpower, *Cambridge, Mass.: Ballinger, 1975. Used with permission.*

in 1978 for $192 billion was very different from and much more valuable than the one bought in 1965 for $43 billion.

Open-heart surgery became a common procedure after the development of the pump-oxygenator, or heart-lung machine, in the late 1950s. By 1976, the annual number of open-heart operations in California alone had reached nearly 15,000, at a cost of roughly $180 million. The coronary artery bypass graft operation—in which a vein from the patient's leg is transplanted to the heart in order to bypass narrowed or blocked segments of the heart's arteries, thereby relieving the chest pain associated with arterial blockage and prolonging the patient's life in some cases—was first done in 1969. By one estimate, at least 70,000 such operations were done in the United States in 1977, at a cost of at least $1 billion.[16]

Intensive-care units for patients with heart attacks and other life-threatening conditions started to become widespread in the late 1950s. Intensive-care units contain systems for monitoring a patient's heart action and other vital signs, as well as life-support systems, including devices that deliver electrical impulses to ailing hearts and machines that maintain patients' breathing. Intensive-care units have been effective in the treatment of various life-threatening illnesses, but they are expensive. Brookings Institution researcher Louise Russell estimated that by 1974, between 4 and 5 percent of all community hospital beds were in intensive-care and coronary-care units.[17] She estimated that average cost per day in these beds was at least three times as high as the cost in an ordinary bed and that the existence of such units raised average hospital cost per day by at least 9 percent, or $10 per day. Multiplied by 260 million days of inpatient care that year would imply an additional cost of $2.6 billion. (Some of the increased cost of these units might be attributed to the extra cost of care of these very sick patients, regardless of the new technology. But the new technology is surely a large contributor to the cost.)

Renal dialysis is the filtering of the blood by artificial kidneys to remove wastes and to maintain the chemical balance of the body. Kidney failure is fatal if untreated. The first dialysis machine was built in the 1940s. Long-term dialysis for chronic kidney failure became practical after 1960, when a device was developed that made it possible to connect the patient to the dialysis machine without surgery for each treatment. In 1972 Congress amended the Social Security Act to extend Medicare coverage to victims of chronic kidney failure. By 1976, this program covered 21,500 eligible patients, at a cost of $448 million. The annual cost of dialysis was estimated at $4500 per patient for home treatment, up to about $30,000 per patient for hospital treatment.[18] In 1977 costs were projected to reach $1.9 billion in 1982.

The late 1960s saw the development of a diagnostic X-ray technology called computerized axial tomography, or C.A.T. scanning. In this technique X-ray beams are projected through the human body from multiple directions, and a computer analyzes the resulting information and reconstructs images of cross-sectional planes. There is no question that the device was a breakthrough in diagnostic technology and has greatly improved the accuracy of diagnosis for certain conditions. It has obviated the need for some exploratory surgery and for some other costly, painful, and sometimes dangerous diagnostic tests. In the mid-1970s most scanners cost from $350,000 to $700,000 to buy and roughly $300,000 per year to operate, with the costs depending on the rate of use. The first unit in the United States was installed in 1973. Some $300 to $400 million was spent on C.A.T. scanning in 1976; by May 1977 at least 400 scanners were in use in the United States.[19]

The list could go on: radiation therapy, total hip and other joint replacements, neonatal intensive care, fetal heart monitoring, and many others. All of this is reflected in such indicators as the increase in hospital employees per patient day from 2.3 in 1960 to 3.4 in 1975. And it has had its effects in many lives saved or greatly improved.

Is the growth in technology a *cause* of the cost increase? Or is it rather a *consequence* of the financial incentives described earlier? The lines of causation are hard to sort out. The invention of a new technology does inspire a demand for its use on the part of those who might be helped by it. Political and social pressures follow to cover it under insurance programs if it is not already covered. This is what occurred, for example, in the case of renal dialysis. The technology came first, then the financing. It is difficult to see how a member of Congress could think that his or her chances for reelection would have been enhanced by a vote against Medicare coverage for renal dialysis in 1972.

But the financial incentives often bias the selection of treatment methods in favor of more costly technologies. For example, one of the main reasons that the costs of the renal-dialysis program have so greatly exceeded their original estimates was the sharp decline in the percentage of patients cared for under the less costly home-dialysis program as compared with those treated in a hospital center. RAND Corporation social scientist Richard Rettig summarized it this way:

> The most obvious factor in the decline of home dialysis, however, is the fact that Medicare law and regulation introduce financial *disincentives* to its use. . . . the method of reimbursing physicians encourages them to treat patients in a center rather than at home, and the patients themselves discover that some of the expenses for which they are not reimbursed at home are covered for patients dialyzed in the center or ·hospital.[20]

Even in cases of cost-reducing technology, such as automated clinical laboratory testing systems, the financial incentives, together with professional and other incentives, have induced such an increase in the use of laboratory tests that the real per capita cost of laboratory tests has increased while the cost per test has been reduced. Thus the problem of cost is not caused by technology as such. Rather, the problem is in the use of technologies in ways that yield little or no health benefit.

From the point of view of public policy, it does not matter much how much of the causation runs which way. There would be no politically possible way of shutting off the development of new medical technology, even if such a course were desirable. If for no other reason, this is so because medical technology is developed in an international marketplace. Few members of Congress would be willing to support a regulatory system that generated news stories of sick people flying to England (where the C.A.T. scanner was first developed) or Holland (where renal dialysis was first developed) to get treatment not available in the United States. But there are politically feasible ways of correcting the financial incentives to reward the use of technology in more cost-effective ways.

Aging Population

Between 1965 and 1978, the number of persons in the United States aged nineteen and under fell from 76.3 million to 71.9 million. The number aged sixty-five and over increased from 18.5 to 24.1 million. Health care costs are much higher for older people. In 1977, for example, personal health expenditures averaged $253 per person under nineteen, $661 per person aged nineteen to sixty-four, and $1745 per person aged sixty-five and over. If we use these expenditures as weights, we can do an approximate calculation of the effect of changing age composition. We assume, hypothetically, that these same per capita expenditures applied in both years, so that the only thing that changed was age composition. (The calculation ignores the large increase in people seventy-five and over, within the sixty-five and over group, and thus produces some understatement of the effect of age.) The result is a 7 percent increase in per capita spending. Thus the age factor, although not insignificant, accounts for a rather small part of the doubling in real per capita spending that took place over these years.

Other Causes

Some people think that too many people go to the doctor unnecessarily and that this is a large contributor to health care costs. There is documentary support for this view. For example, the National Center for Health Statistics reported that a sample of office-based physicians estimated that 48.5 percent of visits were for problems that were not serious. Of course, many of these visits could have been for perfectly good reasons, not at all "unnecessary." The patient might have had no way of knowing that the problem wasn't serious until reassured by the doctor.

It is easy to see how some people could think of unnecessary visits as an important cost factor, especially if their mental picture of the health care system is really the doctor's office. This might be the case for people whose only contact with the system has been the occasional visit to a doctor's office. But it is important to recall that physicians' services account for but 18 percent of the grand total. By one estimate, about 64 percent of the cost of physicians' services is for outpatient services. So even if we estimated that 48.5 percent of visits were unnecessry—an estimate I would consider high—that would mean that only about 6 percent of total health care costs are for unnecessary visits to the doctor. Nevertheless, it would be useful to develop methods of payment that would encourage doctors to instruct their patients in appropriate use of the health care system.

The first cause of rising costs mentioned by many physicians is malpractice suits and the "defensive medicine" that the fear of malpractice suits induces. The existence of malpractice litigation is profoundly distasteful to doctors. Many of them find it an insult to their competence and integrity, random and unfair, and an expression of ingratitude by patients.

What can be said about its effect on costs? The data are poor. Premiums for malpractice insurance, which reflect the costs of litigation and settlements, are not a large part of total health care spending, a few percent at most. Moreover, the part that represents compensation to injured patients for the value of their loss is not a cost to society. The social cost was incurred when they were injured. The costs of "defensive medicine" may be much larger. However, there is no way to measure them. Some practices that are described as defensive medicine may actually be risk-reduction, doing extra tests to reduce the chance of error, something most patients would want done. On the other hand, sometimes the fear of a malpractice suit may decrease the willingness of a physician to undertake a complex, risky procedure. This effect would reduce health care spending. But if the procedure would have helped the patient, the lack of it is a real cost to him. I doubt that any feasible change in our system of malpractice litigation could have a large favorable impact on total health care costs.

ARE DEDUCTIBLES AND COINSURANCE THE SOLUTION?

Since the third-party payment system has so clearly motivated the demanding and providing of more, and more costly, care and the third-party payors have proved to be so powerless to control costs, one wonders what people thought *would* control cost in such a system. One of the main answers is deductibles and coinsurance. Make the patient pay the first $200 of each year's medical bills and 25 percent of the cost above that, and he will be cost-conscious and go to the doctor only when necessary. The doctor, knowing that the patient must pay a quarter of the additional cost of any care he or she prescribes, will then be motivated to be economical in the interest of the patient.

This principle has been applied in most health insurance in the United States. It has formed the basis for an important proposal for national health insurance and cost control by Martin Feldstein of Harvard, called

Major Risk Insurance.[21] The idea appears to be very simple. Let the government provide every family with a comprehensive insurance policy with an annual direct expense limit (a deductible) that is tied to family income. For example, let the direct expense limit be equal to 10 percent of the family's income. The family must pay directly all health care bills, each year, up to the limit. Above the limit, all bills would be paid by insurance. In a more complex version, each family might be required to pay its own medical bills directly until they reached, say, 5 percent of family income. Expenses between 5 and 15 percent of family income would be shared 50-50 with the insurance agency; expenses above 15 percent of family income would be fully paid by insurance. Thus the family's maximum liability would be 10 percent of its income.

These numbers are illustrative. Many variations on the theme are possible. The main idea is to set an expense limit that is high enough so that most bills will be paid directly by individuals, but low enough in relation to family income to prevent serious hardship. The cash-flow problems that this might create for families could be alleviated by government loans. And at least in principle, the scheme could be administered through the personal income tax and cash assistance welfare systems.

This proposal has important strengths. It would prevent financial hardship by limiting each family's health care expenses to 10 percent of income. The fact that most medical bills would be paid directly by patients would reduce the cost of administration and would make consumers cost-conscious. And at least it can be argued that it would lead consumers to seek out cost-conscious doctors, thus putting pressure on all doctors to be economical.

I believe that such heavy reliance on deductibles and coinsurance wouldn't work, even if it could be enacted. And most people show, in their political and market behavior, that they do not like heavy reliance on deductibles and coinsurance. Most of our public and private insurance now has some deductibles and/or coinsurance (though the trend is to reduce both), and that hasn't prevented inflation. It is worth examining why.

First, our society has accepted the principle that everybody should have health insurance of some kind, at least against large expenses. This means that it is inevitable that after spending a certain amount, people will be able to purchase additional amounts of medical care for a price that is either zero or a fraction of their total cost. If the insurance pays 75 percent of bills above the deductible, the consumer still has an incentive to treat a unit of care that costs $20 as if it really cost $5, that is, an incentive to buy "too much." Moreover, in order to protect families from the risk of serious financial loss, an increasing number of insurance policies include an upper limit on the family's out-of-pocket costs, above which all costs will be paid by insurance. This is an essential part of the major-risk insurance idea. At that point, the incentives inherent in the fee-for-service cost-reimbursement, third-party payment system can work their full effect, uninhibited by coinsurance. The effect would be to pull medical resources out of ordinary "primary" care and into the care of "catastrophic" cases, to an extent even greater than occurs today. This would mean less emphasis on activities that can help prevent disease and add significantly to the quality of life and more emphasis on care that offers small or negligible net benefits at very great cost. It would mean a reallocation of health care resources toward categories of care that are probably accounting for too high a share of health care expenditures now. It wouldn't solve the problem of the irrational incentives. It would merely focus them on the most costly cases and forms of care.

Because so much care is elective with respect to timing, much more of it might be done fully paid by major-risk insurance than the proponents of this idea expected. For example, Mrs. Jones was considering having a hysterectomy while Mr. Jones was considering a knee operation. They were discouraged by the fact that they would have to pay for so much of it themselves, until Junior wrapped the family car around a tree and spent a few days in the hospital. That made it a good year in which to have both operations free.

Second, the strategy of reliance on coinsurance assumes, incorrectly, that the purchase of individual units of medical care can be made to be like other normal economic transactions. I believe that it can't be. For most illnesses, the physician cannot quote a fixed price for treatment in advance. You go to the doctor with a pain in your chest and you want to buy a cure. The doctor cannot quote you a price for a cure. Until some diagnostic work has been done, the doctor does not know whether you have indigestion or a heart attack. Once the doctor has made a diagnosis, if the price quoted for further treatment seemed too high, the patient would have to waste much of the money invested in that doctor's services if he wanted to switch doctors to get a lower price. The new doctor would surely want to do his or her own diagnostic tests. Thus in seeking a cure a patient buys a sequence of services whose composition is uncertain at the outset. And the fee for an office visit, for example, may be a very poor indicator of what the total cost for treatment by that doctor will be.

Last spring, Mrs. Smith had no idea that her child would soon come down with pneumonia. So in selecting a pediatrician, she went on the basis of the doctor's fee for a routine follow-up visit and neglected to inquire about the fee for treating a case of pneumonia. How was she to know that the doctor charged $500 for that and ordered three times as many laboratory tests as other doctors would, until she got the bill!

The individual episode of medical care is usually not good material for rational economic calculation. If the patient is in pain or urgent need of care, the transaction is not entirely voluntary. The sick or worried patient is in a poor position to make an economic analysis of treatment alternatives. When my injured child is lying bleeding on the operating table is hardly the time when I want to negotiate with the doctor over fees or the number of sutures that will be used. Of course, not all care is of this urgent nature. There is a whole spectrum, from emergency care for life-threatening conditions to elective cosmetic plastic surgery. One trouble with the major-risk or coinsurance approach is that it applies the same formula across all or most of this spectrum. A better system would rely more heavily on individual judgment in each case.

I believe that the appropriate object for rational economic choice by the consumer is the annual membership in one or another health care plan that provides or pays for comprehensive services (whatever medical care you need) largely for a fixed monthly payment set in advance. (This does not rule out limited use of copayments such as a $5 charge for routine office visits initiated by the patient.) Some of the health care plans that do this are described in Chapter 4. An annual enrollment period is the time when one can reasonably expect most people to make a considered choice. If at that point, the family that chooses a more costly health plan must agree to pay the extra cost out of its own net after-tax income, the family will have a reason to be cost-conscious.

Thus my objection to major-risk insurance is not an objection to making consumers cost-conscious. On the contrary, consumer cost-consciousness is an essential element in any effective solution to the problem of health care costs. My disagreement is over the specific manner in which the element of economic choice is introduced, that is, at the time of medical need rather than at the annual choice of health plan.

Third, it would be very costly for most patients to become well informed about the benefits and costs of alternative treatments. Patients need appropriately motivated doctors to act as their advisors and agents. Comprehensive health care organizations such as those described in Chapter 4 can satisfy this need. Part of what they offer is the confidence that services will be provided only if they are necessary and efficacious.

As noted earlier in this chapter, most Medicare beneficiaries have purchased supplemental private insurance, sometimes called "Medi-gap policies," to fill in the gaps in Medicare coverage. Would this happen under major-risk insurance, and would it defeat the intended incentive effects of the deductibles and coinsurance? What is likely to happen would depend on the way in which the major-risk insurance program and the supplemental private insurance were related to each other. Here the problem begins to get complicated. For example, would the private insurance premium payments be counted as medical expenses toward the family's major-risk deductible? To exclude them—that is to say, that major-risk insurance applies only to direct out-of-pocket payments—would be to bias the system heavily against the purchase of supplemental private insurance and against the purchase of membership in comprehensive health care organizations (see Chapter 4). Even if the beneficiaries were allowed to count their private premium payments as a medical expense for major-risk insurance purposes, the system would be biased against the purchase of private insurance.[22] (Consider two families subject to a $1000 deductible with the same average medical expenses of $800 per year. One pays private-insurance premiums of about $800 per year and never collects from major-risk insurance. The other does not buy private insurance. It has expenses of $200 one year and $1400 the second year. Therefore, it collects $400 from major-risk insurance in the second year and thus collects an average of $200 per year in payments from major-risk insurance. Major-risk insurance favors people with highly variable expenses over those with very regular expenses of the same average amount.)

People who want to use their own money to buy private insurance or to buy membership in a comprehensive-care organization should be treated no less favorably by government than those who do not. Thus an important objective in the design of a government insurance system is neutrality with respect to this choice. That is, on average, government should pay neither more nor less on behalf of similar people who join private health care plans. This is done by offering people who choose private health care plans a fixed payment equal to their expected cost to the government if they did not join a private health care plan, as a premium contribution to the private health plan of their choice. This insight and principle is a foundation of the Consumer Choice Health Plan proposal, described in Chapter 7.

Finally, major-risk insurance ignores the supply side of the medical care market. While trying to make the consumer cost-conscious in the purchase of individual units of care, it leaves the physicians subject to the cost-increasing incentives of fee for service and hospitals paid largely on the basis of costs or cost-based charges. As indicated earlier, it is the physician who makes most of the costly decisions. When they are sick, most people put themselves in the hands of a doctor and ask him or her to take care of them. They don't take out their pocket financial calculators and start to negotiate. Therefore, instead of using the sick patients as the fulcrum for putting leverage on the doctor, it would make much more sense, I believe, to look for modes of organization and payment systems that reward the doctor for cutting cost without cutting the quality of care. How doctors can do this is explained in Chapter 3. Organizations that reward them for doing so are discussed in Chapter 4.

3

Cutting Cost Without Cutting the Quality of Care

A slogan popular among critics of health care cost-containment proposals is: "You can't cut cost without cutting the quality of care or people's access to it." The purpose of this chapter is to show that this slogan is false and seriously misleading as a guide to public policy. It is based on the false assumption that we are now using our health care resources in a way that produces the best possible results for the resources spent. In fact, we are not. There are many ways in which we could achieve large reductions in cost while at the same time *improving*, or at least not reducing, the quality of care. This chapter gives some examples.

REGIONAL CONCENTRATION OF SURGERY AND OTHER SERVICES

Open-Heart Surgery

Stanford doctoral candidate Steven Finkler, C.P.A. and now Ph.D., did a study of the costs of open-heart surgery in California.[1] He spent six months in a large medical center in southern California and developed a complete list of all of the resources used in open-heart surgery. He studied the state regulations and interviewed the physicians and staff in order to develop a detailed picture of the total costs of open-heart surgery. Because different operations have different complexities, he estimated the costs of a representative mix of different types of operations. Then he examined the relationship between the cost per operation and the number of operations performed annually. (His costs include one cardiac catheterization per patient—a diagnostic procedure that precedes open-heart surgery.)

His estimates reflected the actual costs at the number of operations the center was performing and what they would be at different volumes if the same standards were applied. His results are summarized in Fig. 1. He estimated, for example, that the total cost to the system at an annual patient volume of 50 cases was $21,133 per patient in 1976 prices. The cost per patient for 500 cases annually was $8740. Thus major reductions in cost per case are possible when more operations are done at a single facility—a result that would not surprise anyone familiar with industrial economics. The main factor at work is the spreading of fixed costs over a larger number of cases.

Every analysis of this kind must be based on assumptions that might or might not accurately reflect conditions in a particular case. Finkler's analysis assumed that the facilities were dedicated to open-heart surgery and would go unused if not used for that purpose. He also assumed that surgeons not fully occupied with heart surgery filled their schedules with other types of surgery, but that certain technical personnel were fully dedicated to heart surgery. This was the case in the medical center he studied. However, in other medical centers much of the equipment and facilities may be used for other purposes when not used for heart surgery. To the extent that this is the case, the amount of fixed overhead cost associated with heart surgery is reduced, and the curve relating unit cost to number of operations is flatter. On the other hand, more experienced

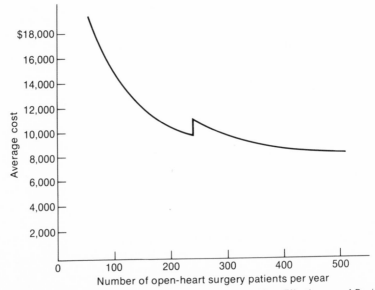

Fig. 1. Average cost for cardiac surgery. [From Steven A. Finkler, "Cost-Effectiveness of Regionalization: The Heart Surgery Example." Reprinted, with permission of the Blue Cross Association, from Inquiry **16**, *3 (Fall 1979): 266. Copyright © 1979 by the Blue Cross Association. All rights reserved.]*

heart-surgery units are likely to produce better results (see below). Proficiency should mean less time in the operating room and shorter lengths of hospital stay for patients. Unfortunately, we do not have data on the last two points. But these factors would increase the savings associated with volume. Pending the availability of more data and analysis, I accept Finkler's curve as a good approximation of the actual situation.

Finkler went on to ask where heart surgery was being done in California and at what volumes. He found that 14,835 operations were being performed in ninety-one hospitals, for an average of 163 per hospital. Of the ninety-one hospitals, fifty-nine, or 65 percent of the total, were doing fewer than 150 operations per year, forty-eight were doing fewer than 100. Only eleven were doing more than 300 per year. He calculated the hypothetical annual costs of open-heart surgery in the state, assuming that each hospital's cost per patient was the same as it would have been in the hospital he studied, but at its respective volume. The state total was $180 million. Then he calculated what the costs would have been if instead, all of the operations had been done at thirty medical centers, each doing about 500 per year. That came to $136 million. Thus he calculated that $44 million per year, or 24 percent of the total costs, could have been saved by concentrating open-heart surgery in thirty regional centers.

What about quality? The fact that so many hospitals were doing fewer than 150 operations per year—indeed fewer than 100 in more than half of the centers—is particularly significant because the various specialty societies for the most part recommend minimum volumes of 150 or 200 cases per year in order to maintain proficiency. For example, the American Heart Association recommended a minimum volume of at least 150 operations per year; the American College of Surgeons, 100 to 150 per team; the Inter-Society Commission for Heart Disease Resources, at least 200.

Two of my Stanford colleagues, economist Harold Luft, Ph.D., and John Bunker, M.D., and I did a study of the relationship between the percentage of surgery patients dying in the hospital and annual volume (while statistically controlling for case severity), for twelve operations done in nearly 1500 hospitals in 1974 and 1975.[2] One of the categories of operations was open-heart surgery, and our findings are summarized in Fig. 2. We found, for example, that the average death rate at an annual volume of 50 operations was about 11.5 percent, whereas in hospitals doing 300 operations per year, it was about 6.5 percent. Put alternatively, we found that the hospitals where fewer than 200 operations were done per year had death rates 24 percent above the average for the mix of patients they treated. The hospitals where more than 200 operations were done had death rates 23 percent below the average. In our sample of 27,471 patients, 2228 died. If instead, the results obtained in the low-volume hospitals had been as good as those obtained in the high-volume hospitals, there would have been 492, or 22 percent, fewer deaths. Of course, this is a hypothetical

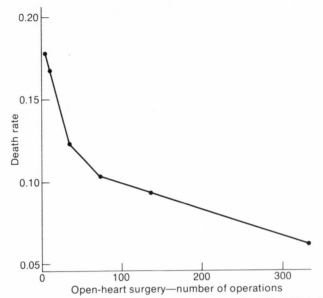

Fig. 2. *Relationship between death rate and number of operations.* [*From Harold S. Luft, John P. Bunker, and Alain C. Enthoven, "Should Operations Be Regionalized? The Empirical Relation Between Surgical Volume and Mortality." Reprinted by permission from the* New England Journal of Medicine **301**, *25 (December 20, 1979): 1366.*]

statement. We found a statistically significant relationship between volume and death rate, but we did not prove the existence of a cause-and-effect relationship.

The explanation of the relationship between volume and the mortality rate is a complex matter. I believe that a substantial part of the explanation is the "experience effect." That is, the quality of care improves with the experience of those providing it. Hospitals and surgical teams that perform many operations maintain high proficiency, correcting the sources of error in their techniques. "Learning by doing" is a common phenomenon and is the basis for much of medical education. Great surgeons, like great artists and great athletes, are at their best when they practice regularly. Presumably, the specialty societies and commissions accept this explanation when they recommend that volumes should not be below minimum guideline levels. However, there are alternative explanations. One is simply that hospitals that do a better job attract more patients. In other words, the causality runs from better results to more patients, rather than vice versa. It is also possible that the high-volume hospitals treat patients who are less likely to die. We applied the best available statistical measure to control for this factor and found that it did not explain away our results. The relative significance of these factors remains uncertain.

If we accept that a higher volume of operations leads to a lower death rate, the implication is clear. Californians undergoing open-heart surgery would get much better care at much lower cost if heart surgery were done at thirty regional centers rather than at the current ninety-one hospitals. Rather than lower costs meaning lower quality, this is one example of a change that would produce lower costs while producing better quality.

Maternity

Ann Pettigrew, M.D., M.P.H., with the Massachusetts Department of Public Health, studied maternity and newborn care in Massachusetts and recommended a regional organization of these services.[3] The idea was that the goals of both quality and economy could be served best if deliveries and intensive care of newborn infants were concentrated in hospitals with enough cases to maintain the proficiency of the specialized personnel. She recommended immediately closing all maternity units with fewer than 500 deliveries a year (except for a few geographically isolated cases), twenty-seven out of seventy-five units in 1975, and ultimately establishing a minimum standard of 1500 deliveries for urban hospitals. Only fourteen of seventy-five units met this standard in 1975. (This could be done without significant increases in travel times for patients.) In addition, she recommended a statewide system of maternity units at three levels of care: (1) uncomplicated deliveries plus minimum capabilities for stabilizing unexpected emergencies, prior to transportation; (2) intermediate capabilities; and (3) a full range of specialized maternal, fetal, and newborn services. The study did not report total statewide cost estimates for the existing system compared with the recommended system. But one indication of the possible economies available is that the costs of an efficient minimum-capability maternity unit would have been $1245 per admission at 500 admissions per year, compared with only $653 per admission at 1200 admissions per year (1975 prices).

Other Services

The same principles apply to other types of surgery and medical care. Luft, Bunker, and I found results similar to those for open-heart surgery in the case of operations on blood vessels, prostate, and for total hip replacement. However, some operations, such as removal of the gallbladder, showed no experience effect on the death rate. As one would expect, the experience effect appears to be related to the complexity of the procedure.

The same economies of scale are available in other services for which there are large fixed costs: radiation therapy, clinical laboratories, and C.A.T. scanning. Thus viewing the medical care system as a whole, we could realize substantial improvements in quality and cost if we had a system that responded to these opportunities. In Chapters 4 and 5 I will describe how such a system might be created.

MATCHING RESOURCES USED TO THE NEEDS OF THE POPULATION SERVED

These examples illustrate a general principle of health care economics. The goals of proficiency and economy are best served when the numbers and types of physicians in a community are matched to the needs of the population served in such a way that each specialist is kept fully occupied seeing patients who require his or her special expertise. More than that number of doctors will mean unnecessarily higher cost and reduced proficiency. It may also mean more care yielding little or no benefit to patients. Similarly, proficiency and economy are best served when the supply of hospital beds and specialized facilities is matched to the needs of the population served. Excess beds and facilities add to cost without adding to the quality of care.

Let me use some of the findings described in Chapter 2 to construct a hypothetical example that illustrates the point about physician supply. The numbers are chosen to be roughly representative of the situation in 1979. Consider two similar communities of 100,000 people each, one served by ten general surgeons kept fully occupied with general surgery and the other served by twenty. Assume that the gross revenue of a general surgeon is $120,000 a year. The first community has a per capita cost of $12 per year for general surgeons and ten proficient surgeons. If the surgeons in the second community follow the pattern found by Uwe Reinhardt, described in Chapter 2, they will do what they need to do to make their $120,000, that is, charge higher fees and do more surgery. If the surgeons in the second community follow the pattern found by Victor Fuchs, described in Chapter 2, they will do thirty percent more operations. (A 30 percent increase in surgery associated with a 100 percent increase in the number of surgeons is equivalent to a three percent increase in surgery associated with a ten percent increase in the number of surgeons.) Suppose further that in the first community, each surgeon does 500 operations per year and that hospital costs average $2000 per case. Then the citizens in this community will undergo 5000 operations at a cost per capita for general surgery of $112. The citizens in the second community will undergo 6500 operations at a cost per capita for general surgery of $154. Surgeons in this community will average 325 operations a year.

This example illustrates how more doctors can lead to more cost and to less busy doctors. It does not show that the larger number of doctors and operations yields no additional health benefit. It might or might not, depending on the circumstances. (See the next section for a discussion of this.) But if the citizens really do benefit from 6500 instead of 5000 operations, the example does imply that they could get them at less cost and from more proficient surgeons if they retained thirteen surgeons, each doing 500 operations, instead of twenty surgeons.

I believe that this example tells the story of what is happening in an increasing number of communities and specialities in the United States.

While some areas remain underserved, others are getting too many doctors, and the extra services they are providing are not contributing to improved health. Admittedly, this must be a matter of judgment because we do not have standards for the appropriate number of doctors.

The root of the problem of too many doctors in some communities is that the insured fee-for-service system is very permissive with respect to physician decisions about location and specialty. Most people have to live near where they can find a job. But physicians have a great deal of freedom to set up practice in areas they find attractive for living. New doctors who want to practice in an area that already has too many doctors can do so and still make an adequate living because the fees there will be higher and they can recommend more of their services to insured patients. The doctors in excess supply are under economic pressure to find ways to make themselves useful, and insured patients have weak financial incentives to question the value of the services. The economic disincentives to practicing in an attractive but oversupplied area are often not strong enough to overcome the attractions. All this stands in sharp contrast to the practices of organized systems that care for enrolled populations. They do control the number of physicians and match them to the needs of the populations they serve.

Any specific numerical comparison is hazardous, because the physicians in a particular county may serve patients living in a wider area. Also, some services may be provided about equally well by physicians of different specialities. And there may be significant differences in the medical needs of different populations, for example because of age. So any example will inspire endless arguments. Still, I believe that we have too many doctors in San Francisco. Table 1 compares the number of physicians

TABLE 1   Physicians in Office-Based Patient Care per 100,000 Population

	San Francisco 1975[a]	California 1975[b]	United States 1977[c]	Kaiser-Permanente 1975[d]
Dermatology	6.0	2.7	1.8	2.9
Ophthalmology	13.6	5.4	4.3	3.2
Neurosurgery	3.7	1.4	1.0	.6
Total	292.6	138.8	106.5	105.2

[a] *Numerators used by permission from* Characteristics of Physicians, California, *American Medical Association, December 31, 1975. Denominator from* Population Projections for California Counties 1975–2020, Sacramento: Population Research Unit, Department of Finance, State of California, December 1977. (7-1-75 population.)
[b] *Numerators from L. J. Goodman and H. R. Mason,* Physician Distribution and Medical Licensure in the U.S., 1975. Center for Health Services Research and Development. Chicago: American Medical Association, 1976. Denominator same as [a]. Data used by permission.*
[c] *Department of Statistical Analysis,* Physician Distribution and Medical Licensure in the U.S., 1977. Center for Health Services Research and Development. Chicago: American Medical Association, 1979. (12-31-1977 resident population.) Data used by permission.*
[d] *Kaiser-Permanente Medical Care Program, Northern California Region.*

in office-based patient care per 100,000 population in San Francisco with the numbers in California, the United States, and in the Kaiser-Permanente Medical Care Program in northern California.[4] The Kaiser program, an example of what is known as a prepaid group practice, now serves more than 3.5 million people and is described in Chapter 4. Although there is no basis for saying that the Kaiser program has the "right" number of doctors, it does have an incentive to employ what is, in its judgment, an appropriate number. If the program employs too many, its costs will increase; if it employs too few, its enrolled members (and the doctors) will be dissatisfied. Either way, the program's ability to compete in the marketplace would be weakened. San Francisco has about three times the per capita number of doctors in office-based patient care as the nation as a whole or as the Kaiser program and about three times in some specialties, such as ophthalmology. This helps to explain why the Medicare reimbursement for physician services per person enrolled in 1977 in San Francisco was 43 percent above the national average.

From 1960 to 1975, the number of short-term general hospital beds per 1000 people in the United States increased from 3.6 to 4.5. This stands in sharp contrast to the 1.5 to 1.6 beds per 1000 required by organized systems such as Kaiser-Permanente and Group Health Cooperative of Puget Sound. Part of the difference can be accounted for by differences in the average age of the populations served. If Kaiser and Group Health served a representative mix of population, they would need some 1.8 to 2 beds per 1000. Most of the difference, however, can be accounted for by the fact that doctors outside these organized systems (the fee-for-service sector) hospitalize equivalent patients more.

The percentage of beds occupied is also a factor. The California Health Facilities Commission staff estimated that in 1976 the average occupancy rate for Kaiser hospitals in California was about 81 percent of available beds, compared with 64 percent in northern California and 61 percent in southern California for non-Kaiser hospitals.[5] The reason for this difference is that the ordinary community hospital can pass on its costs to third parties and has little or no financial incentive to avoid excess capacity. In other words, being only 64 percent occupied poses no serious problem. In fact, the management of these hospitals are not likely to have a clear idea of what populations they do serve. On the other hand, hospital-based prepaid group practice plans such as Kaiser and Group Health Cooperative have a financial incentive to match carefully their facilities to the needs of the populations they serve. And they do serve a defined enrolled population. If they build a hospital that is not needed, they will have to pay for it themselves anyway out of the fixed monthly contributions of their enrolled members. They cannot pass it on to third parties. This helps explain why the hospital expense per person cared for in one of these systems is so much lower than it is for similar people cared for in the fee-for-service sector.

CURTAILING "FLAT-OF-THE-CURVE MEDICINE"

Diminishing Marginal Returns Explained

On a certain piece of farm land, ten workers produce 50,000 bushels of grain. Add another worker, and the yield goes up to 54,000 bushels, for an increase of 4000 bushels. Add still another worker, and the yield goes up to 57,000 bushels, for an increase of 3000 bushels. Eventually, the addition of yet another worker adds nothing to the yield.

Add a salesman to a certain territory, and sales go up by $100,000. Add another, and sales go up an additional $80,000. Eventually, the addition of yet another salesman to the territory adds nothing to the total sales.

For a seriously ill patient, the first day in the hospital is clearly beneficial. The next few days are as well, though perhaps each one makes less difference to the patient's health status than the day before did. Eventually, there comes a time when an additional day in the hospital will yield no benefit at all.

These are examples of "the law of diminishing marginal returns," a basic principle of economics. As an empirical generalization, this law fits many (though not all) situations in the production of goods and services and in such areas as national defense and environmental protection, as well as medical care.

This principle is illustrated in Fig. 3; a health benefit is measured on the vertical axis, and dollar cost or some other measure of resources used is measured on the horizontal axis. As drawn here, eventually the curve becomes flat (no more benefits are obtained) as more resources are applied, hence the expression "flat-of-the-curve medicine." Of course, the curve might not become flat. It might keep on rising slowly, as, for example, in

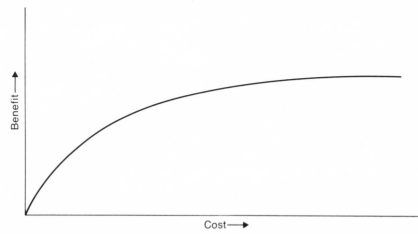

Fig. 3. Diminishing marginal returns.

the case of repeated applications of a test, each of which slightly improves the likelihood that a diagnosis is correct. Or, it might actually turn down, as is suggested by the examples in Chapter 1 in which more medical care is actually harmful. Whether or not the extra benefits at any point are worth the extra costs is, or course, a matter of judgment about the value of the extra benefits and of the other benefits that might be obtained by the use of those resources.

I believe that a great deal of "flat-of-the-curve medicine" is being practiced in the United States today—that health care resources are being used in ways that yield very little or no discernible health benefit.

Wide Variations in Per Capita Use of Services, with No Discernible Difference in Health

In Chapter 1 we saw that Dr. Paul Lembcke observed wide variations in the per capita rate of appendectomies in different hospital service areas of New York and found that fewer operations for appendicitis did not mean higher appendicitis death rates. If anything, he found the opposite. His data suggest that patients in areas where many appendectomies were performed would have been better off if the number of operations per capita had been reduced to that in the areas with a low rate.

More recently, John Wennberg, M.D., of Harvard Medical School, and Alan Gittelsohn, Ph.D., a Johns Hopkins biostatistician, found wide variations in the per capita use of various health services in thirteen different service areas of Vermont, despite the similarity of the populations in terms of rates of illness, income, racial and social background, insurance coverage, and number of physician visits per capita.[6] They found that the overall per capita rate of surgical operations in some areas was twice that in others (after adjusting the comparison to take account of difference in the age and sex compositions of the populations), with much wider variations for some operations. For example, they found rates of tonsillectomy varying from four to forty-one per 1000 children per year. Rates of hysterectomy ranged from thirty to sixty per 10,000 women per year. There was also wide variation in the use of other types of care. For example, among Medicare enrollees, total laboratory services per capita varied by 700 percent. Commenting on the effects of medical care on those living in the high-cost areas, Dr. Wennberg observed, "There is no evidence that the latter have greater medical need, or indeed that more health is produced . . . in terms of their health status, it is not possible in my opinion to argue that Vermonters in more expensive areas are better or worse for the effort."[7] Other studies have documented similar variations elsewhere.

Length of Hospital Stay for Heart Attack Patients

Dr. Adolph Hutter and his colleagues at Massachusetts General Hospital did a study of early hospital discharge after myocardial infarction (heart attack).[8] They evaluated patients on the sixth day in the hospital as "complicated" or "uncomplicated." The "uncomplicated" were randomly assigned to either a two- or a three-week total hospital stay. During the six-month follow-up period, there was no difference between the two- and the three-week patients in frequency of return to work, anxiety or depression, heart condition, or survival. "There appears to be no additional benefit to the patient with an uncomplicated myocardial infarction from a three-week as compared to a two-week hospital stay."[9] In a more recent study, doctors at Duke University tried sending home half of the patients on the seventh day and found similar results.[10] And, as described in Chapter 1, British studies have shown that for many (but not all) uncomplicated heart attack patients, hospitalization produces no discernible advantage, compared with home care, for the patient's health.

There were more than 380,000 hospital admissions for acute myocardial infarction in the United States in 1974. The average length of stay was 14.4 days. So patients with this diagnosis accounted for about 5.5 million hospital days. During later days in a hospital stay, services are used less intensively than during earlier days, so an overall average cost per day can give only a very rough indicator of potential savings. Nevertheless, at about $190 per day in 1978 dollars, the savings that could be realized from cutting this length of stay in half might have exceeded $400 million per year.

Second Opinions for Surgery

Another indication of "flat-of-the-curve medicine" is provided by the results of second-opinion surgical-consultation programs such as the one directed by Eugene G. McCarthy, M.D., of Cornell University Medical College, for several unions in New York.[11] In some of the programs a second opinion was voluntary; in others, mandatory. In the voluntary programs 34 percent of the recommendations for surgery were not confirmed by the second opinion. In the mandatory program 17 percent of the recommendations were not confirmed. (The percentage is higher in the voluntary programs because the people who choose to get second opinions are likely to be in doubt about the need for surgery.) In some specialties, such as orthopaedics and gynecology, the percentage of recommendations for surgery not confirmed by second opinion was much higher.

I like to avoid the term "unnecessary surgery" in discussing such findings, although that term will inevitably be used in some circles. I am quite prepared to believe that in most of the cases not confirmed by a second opinion, the patient had a real ailment to which the recommended operation was addressed. Moreover, I believe that most physicians sincerely want to do the best thing for their patients and that the surgeons recommending these operations honestly believed that they were acting in the best interest of their patients. John Bunker, M.D., and Byron Brown,

Jr., Ph.D., of Stanford Medical School did a study comparing per capita rates of surgery for physicians and their spouses with those for other professionals and their families.[12] They found that operation rates for physicians and spouses were as high as or higher than for other groups. These findings support the view that physicians believe in what they are recommending. Moreover, in some cases it may cost as much to treat the patient without surgery as with surgery, so that avoiding surgery may not save much money. But these second-opinion results do suggest that in many cases, the risks and benefits to the patient are quite closely balanced. If two surgeons, both well qualified and honestly seeking what is best for the patient, come to different conclusions about the advisability of an operation, generally speaking the net benefits, compared with some other course of treatment, must not be large or obvious. One might say that some of the operations are examples of "flat-of-the-curve" medical care.

Electronic Fetal Monitoring

Another example of "flat-of-the-curve medicine" may be in the use of electronic fetal monitoring. In this procedure electronic instruments are passed into the uterus and are attached to the fetus at the beginning of the birth process. The purpose is to detect fetal distress which, if uncorrected, might threaten brain damage or death. Detection of distress may lead to a decision to deliver by Caesarian section. As a consequence, the percentage of deliveries by Caesarian section has increased from 5.5 in 1965 to 12.5 in 1976. All this has risks, including injuries to the fetal scalp, infection, fetal distress induced by the monitoring, and the risks of surgery associated with Caesarian section. By one estimate, monitoring in the mid-1970s added some $35 to $75 to the cost of delivery, while Caesarian section raised the hospital cost of delivery from $700 to $3000.[13]

Raymond Neutra, M.D., then of Harvard Medical School, and his colleagues did an analysis of 15,846 live-born infants to assess the effect of electronic monitoring on newborn death rates.[14] They developed a numerical risk score based on eighteen factors believed to influence the likelihood of death of newborn infants, including, for example, number of weeks of pregnancy, single or multiple birth, position of the fetus, race, and mother's age. They classified all of the births into five risk categories and compared the death rates for those monitored and those not monitored in each category. They found that in the 0.76 percent of the births in the highest-risk category, monitoring was associated with a reduction in death rate from 303.8 to 195.1 per 1000 births. In the 76.1 percent of the births in the lowest-risk category, the death rate per 1000 was 0.5 for those *not* monitored and 1.1 for those who were. That is, in the low-risk deliveries, monitoring apparently does more harm than good. Their results are summarized in Table 2.

As Dr. Neutra pointed out, the research design of the study and the statistical results left room for doubt. (It was not a randomized trial, and

TABLE 2   Effect of Fetal Monitoring on Neonatal Death Rates within Strata of Risk

Risk-Score Category	Percent of Sample in Category	Monitored?	Death Rates Per 1000	Differences in Death Rates
Highest risk	0.76	No	303.8	108.7
		Yes	195.1	
High	0.73	No	80.7	43.0
		Yes	37.7	
Medium	3.80	No	20.7	5.9
		Yes	14.8	
Low	18.60	No	5.2	2.7
		Yes	2.5	
Lowest	76.10	No	0.5	−0.6
		Yes	1.1	

Source: Raymond R. Neutra et al., "Effect of Fetal Monitoring on Neonatal Death Rates," New England Journal of Medicine **299** (August 17, 1978): 324–326. Used with permission.

the possibility that the results were produced by chance or some factor other than monitoring could not be ruled out.) Nevertheless, if one takes the numbers at face value, they make an interesting point. If one monitors only the highest-risk groups, the total costs are small and the benefits substantial. If one monitors the whole population, the costs are very large, and the benefits obtained from monitoring the majority who are in the lowest-risk category are small, possibly negative. The key issue, then, is not "monitor everybody or nobody"; it is "how far down the risk scale should we monitor?"

The Need for Benefit-Cost Analysis

"Flat-of-the-curve" medicine appears sometimes to occur because of a lack of careful analysis of all of the costs, risks, and benefits associated with a procedure. A new technology is developed, is found to be apparently efficacious in some cases, and then is applied to many cases before a careful study is done. David Eddy, M.D., Ph.D., a Stanford professor who applies detailed mathematical analysis to clincial policies, did a study, including a thorough review of the medical literature through 1975, of the clincial policy-making process in mammography (X-ray of the breast to detect cancer).[15] Among other problems, he found numerous errors in probability reasoning and a general pattern of single-minded pursuit of breast-cancer detection to the exclusion of other relevant considerations such as the "false-positive rate" (how often the test says the woman has cancer when in fact she doesn't) and the costs, risks, and discomfort of biopsies (surgical removal of breast tissue for microscopic examination) performed because of false positive results, X-ray radiation hazards, and the monetary costs of the procedure. Such single-minded reasoning was at the basis of many recommendations to use mammography annually to screen relatively young, symptom-free women, for whom the probability of cancer is extremely low and for whom the net benefit of the test is very doubtful.

"Benefit-cost analysis," sometimes called "cost-effectiveness analysis," is a fairly recent development in medical care. It is a synthesis of principles of economics, statistics, probability, and decision theory applied to the complex and uncertain problems of medical decision making. The goal is to elucidate all of the costs, risks, and benefits of alternative courses of action so that decision makers can be well informed in applying the necessary judgments. Such analysis, properly conceived, should be an aid to judgment, not a substitute for it. Analytical aids to decision making have been developed and applied extensively in such fields as industrial management, natural-resource development, environmental protection, and national defense. I believe that benefit-cost analysis has great potential for aiding physicians who want to cut cost without cutting the quality of care.

A Consumer- versus Provider-Oriented Concept of Quality

There are many cases in which the curve relating benefits to costs will not be absolutely flat. There may be small gains in detection probabilities and life expectancy (and also large costs) from more frequently repeated application of diagnostic screening tests. Dr. Eddy has estimated, for example, that increasing the frequency of Pap smears from every two years to every year for a woman of average risk, starting at age twenty-five, will add about 2.5 days to her life expectancy at an additional cost of about $86 (measured in present value of the projected cost over the patient's lifetime). An increase in the frequency of mammograms from every two years to every year for a woman of average risk, starting at age fifty, will add about nine days to her life expectancy at an additional cost of about $500.[16] Who is to say that $500 is too much or that the frequency should be increased even more?

One point of view defines the best quality of care as the maximum that medical care can do to prolong life or alleviate suffering, costs not considered. According to this view, any level of care short of the point at which no more benefit is produced is less than optimum care. A decision to provide such an amount, rather than more care, is a reduction in quality. This is a professionally oriented concept of quality. It is the concept that many people have in mind when they say: "You can't cut cost without cutting the quality of care."

I believe that this is not a valid concept of quality, however. People do not act in such a way as to maximize their life expectancy in other dimensions of their lives, so why should they in choices of medical care? They drive cars, fly in airplanes, cross streets, climb mountains, not to mention smoke and drink excessively. And they willingly undergo surgery intended simply to improve the quality of their lives, even at some risk of dying from the operation. So there is no reason to think that they would want to or should use medical services to the extent that they yield the last possible small increase in life expectancy. There are other than financial costs that people want to avoid, including time costs and the unpleasantness of treatment. People's preferences for risk reductions, compared with the benefits they would receive from other uses of the resources, ought to be considered. Some risk reductions are not worth having at the cost. Even from the point of view of health, at some point dollars are better spent on other things, such as food and housing, rather than on more medical care. Some terminal patients may not want a few more days or weeks of suffering life.

The best quality care is not that care which ekes out the last possible day of life expectancy. Rather, the best quality of care reflects society's preferences in the use of resources. It is being provided when the extra health benefits yielded by expenditure of another dollar of resources on medical care are valued by consumers the same as they value the benefits obtained from the same expenditure in other activities, that is, when medical spending and other spending are in balance.

THE CONTROLLED INTRODUCTION OF NEW TECHNOLOGY

The history of medicine includes many innovations that were initially greeted with enthusiasm and then subsequently dropped for lack of evidence that they were beneficial to the patient.[17] For example, before the introduction of the coronary artery bypass graft operation, described below, five different operations were developed for coronary artery disease, widely accepted, and then later abandoned. New drugs can be introduced for general use only after proof of their efficacy based on thorough testing in carefully designed experiments. But new technologies often move quickly into widespread application without the benefit of similar evaluation. Only a small minority of medical innovations are tested by a randomized clinical trial before they are put into widespread application.[18]

Physician innovators are often very enthusiastic about the new procedures they invent, much more so when their evaluations are not based on controlled trials than when they are. And many innovations prove not to be preferred to standard existing treatment when evaluated by a randomized clinical trial. (Of course, there may be a bias in the selection of procedures to be evaluated. Only those whose efficacy is in controversy or doubt may be evaluated.)

There are many conceptual and practical difficulties that must be surmounted in planning and executing a good randomized clinical trial. And even well-designed trials do not answer all of the important questions or settle all of the arguments. Scientific evaluation of the efficacy of medical treatment can be an extremely complex and difficult matter. Nevertheless, I believe that many more innovations should be evaluated by this means. In any case, innovations in medical technology should be thoroughly evaluated early, before being put into widespread use, especially if they involve large sums of money.

A spectacular example of the need for such evaluation before widespread use is coronary artery bypass graft surgery as a treatment for coronary artery disease. This disease can lead to severe chest pain (angina pectoris) and/or myocardial infarction. Millions of Americans suffer from coronary artery disease. It can be treated "medically," that is, with drugs, diet, and exercise, or surgically. Bypass graft surgery was first introduced in the late 1960s, and it spread rapidly. About 25,000 such operations were done in 1973, more than 70,000 in 1977. At about $15,000 per operation, the Office of Technology Assessment estimated an annual cost of over $1 billion for this one operation in 1977.

In the early 1970s, the Veterans Administration conducted a randomized clinical trial at thirteen of its hospitals, with more than 1000 patients, roughly half of whom were treated medically, the other half surgically. Surgical treatment was found to be beneficial for one type of patient. About eleven percent of the patients had diseased left main coronary arteries. In this group the patients treated surgically had a significantly better survival rate than did those treated medically. As for the others, there was no statistically significant difference in survival between the two groups at follow-ups twenty-one and thirty-six months after entry into the trial. At the end of thirty-six months, 87 percent of the group treated medically and 88 percent of the group treated surgically were alive.[19] Thus by the time the full results of the first large-scale randomized clinical trial were published, a $1 billion-a-year industry had been created and was firmly in place.

The report of the study triggered a stormy debate. I believe that such debate is very healthy. The value of this surgery is still in question, and the debate helps to clarify the issues, which are very complex. But I also believe that it would have been better if the operation had been limited to perhaps a few thousand per year and done in a few centers under carefully designed experimental protocols until it was clearly established which, if any, patients would benefit from it. Such an approach would have led to better care (including fewer deaths from the operation) at a substantially lower cost.

A similar point can be made with respect to computerized axial tomography. As mentioned in Chapter 2, the first installation in the United States took place in 1973. The Office of Technology Assessment estimated that the gross annual expenditures on C.A.T. scanning in 1976 were somewhere between $293 and $426 million; the net, after subtraction of costs of tests it replaced, at some $180 to $388 million.[20] All of this took place in the absence of any established guidelines for use of C.A.T.[21]

There is no evidence that Americans would not be just as healthy with half as many scanners. Again, early controlled evaluations leading to guidelines for use of this technology might have saved a great deal of money.

Physicians should forebear in the widespread diffusion of costly new technology until some kind of thorough evaluation has been done. John Bunker, University of Minnesota statistician David Hinkley, Ph.D., and W. V. McDermott, M.D., of Harvard Medical School, recommended the creation of an "Institute of Health Care Assessment" to provide an independent evaluation of surgical procedures, to act as a "central reviewing authority capable of sophisticated statistical and economic analysis and empowered with authority and resources necessary to initiate and coordinate appropriate trials."[22] Similar evaluation of other new technologies and of many existing practices is needed. I believe that it would be better if this were done on a private and voluntary basis by the medical profession rather than by the government.

SIMPLE COST CONSCIOUSNESS

Equivalent Care in Less Costly Sites

There is a great deal of routine, nonemergency physician care that is delivered in hospital emergency rooms in inner cities because care in physicians' offices is not available. Emergency rooms cost much more to build and to operate than do ordinary physicians' offices. Outpatient, or "same day," surgery has grown in importance in recent years. Many cases that could be treated this way are still treated on a more costly inpatient basis.

The British studies of home versus hospital care for patients suspected of having acute myocardial infarction point to another area of large potential savings. That is, medically equivalent results can be achieved in some cases at substantially less cost through organized home care instead of hospital care. One study of stroke patients in New York found lower costs and better results in a group discharged from the hospital earlier and supported by organized home care, compared with another group hospitalized longer and not given home care.[23] Groups in the United States and the United Kingdom have developed similar home-care support services as an alternative to long-term institutionalization for the elderly.[24] There is excessive use of hospital instead of home care because the third-party payors often will pay for the former, but not for the support services required for the latter. Also, health professionals in general are biased in favor of institutional care. Yet home care may offer substantial advantages in appropriately selected cases.

Duplicate Tests, Excessive Hospital Stays, Sheer Waste

The foregoing are relatively subtle notions—forms of waste that are not obvious, one might say. There is also a great deal of obvious waste. Many people are admitted to the hospital for diagnostic workups that could be performed equally well at lower cost on an outpatient basis. Other people receive tests on an inpatient basis that duplicate those that led to the decision to hospitalize them, often because the hospital management wants to generate more revenue for its laboratory and X-ray departments. (Blue Cross has recently announced that it will no longer pay for this.) Wide variations in length of stay for the same diagnosis and treatment suggest that many stays could be greatly reduced with no loss in quality of medical outcome. And the existence of such waste is widely recognized by professionals in the field. The problem is that under our predominant system of organization and finance, waste is supported, and there are no incentives for economy. If we want to see economical behavior, we must look to the alternative health care financing and delivery systems that are the subject of the next chapter.

4

Alternative Financing and Delivery Systems

THE HMO ACT AND THE IDEA OF ALTERNATIVE DELIVERY SYSTEMS

What are the alternatives to insured fee for service? If it is possible to cut cost without cutting the quality of care, how can medical care be organized to encourage this? If there are organizations that use health care resources economically, what can be done to encourage their growth?

This chapter reviews the alternatives to insured fee for service. It explains how some of the alternative systems are organized to encourage economy. Chapter 5, on economic competition among health care financing and delivery systems, explains what can be done to encourage their growth.

Paul M. Ellwood, M.D., president of InterStudy, a research and policy analysis institute devoted to health care and located near Minneapolis, is, in my view, one of the most creative thinkers on the national health care scene. In 1970 he and several of his associates proposed a national "Health Maintenance Strategy" based on competing private comprehensive health care organizations, which they called "health maintenance organizations," or "HMOs."[1] He sold the idea to the Secretary of Health, Education, and Welfare, and it was embraced briefly by the Nixon administration. The idea attracted support in the Congress, where Congressman William R. Roy, M. D., and Senator Edward M. Kennedy introduced legislation intended to encourage the development of HMOs. The admirers and the enemies of the concept teamed up to define HMOs in very ambitious terms. The former sought to make them embody their dreams of the perfect health care delivery system, whereas the latter sought to make them so costly that they would be unable to compete effectively with traditional insurance plans, which are not required to meet the same criteria. The result was a detailed and narrow definition of an HMO—including a generous list of covered benefits, pricing and enrollment practices, physician organization, and requirements regarding assumption of financial risk.

Many of the organizations that would have fit nicely into Ellwood's original concept and strategy did not find themselves described accurately in the Health Maintenance Organization Act of 1973. Fortunately, the law was amended in 1976 to eliminate some of the most costly provisions. Because of the unnecessary detail in the legal definition of an HMO, Ellwood, in collaboration with an associate, Walter McClure, Ph.D., then sought a broader term. They have subsequently referred to "alternative health care financing and delivery systems," or "alternative delivery systems."[2] The main principles defining an alternative delivery system are the following.

First, in the insured fee-for-service system, *premiums are paid to a financial intermediary.* After care has been given, the patient or the provider sends the bill to the patient's intermediary. More, and more costly, services mean more revenue to the providers. This creates a problem of excessive cost because consumers depend on providers for advice on the need for services, and insured consumers have little or no reason to consider the cost of the services they receive.

In an alternative delivery system, *premiums are paid to an organization that itself accepts responsibility for providing or arranging comprehensive services.* The premium is set in advance on the basis of a fixed amount per person per month. This premium must cover all or nearly all of the cost of whatever services are necessary. Thus the provider organization has a fixed budget within which to provide the care. More services do not mean more revenue.

Second, in the insured fee-for-service system, *the patient has "free choice of doctor."* (I put this in quotes because in fact, the patient is limited in his choice by many factors, including the willingness of doctors to accept him as a patient, his limited knowledge about other doctors, dependence on one doctor for referrals to another, and distance. "Free choice of doctor" means that the insurance policy does not place any limit on the choice of licensed doctors.) Because the costs associated with one patient are generally small in relation to the total costs for the insured group, the patient's premium payment is virtually the same whichever providers he chooses. There is thus little or no incentive to choose an economical doctor. Economical providers are not rewarded with more patients. The system precludes economic competition among providers.

In an alternative delivery system, *the patient accepts a limited choice of doctors, including only those participating in that particular system,* in exchange for what he perceives to be better benefits or lower costs. The patient is usually free to choose a doctor from among those in the organization, and if given a free choice of alternative delivery systems, he may join the system with his favorite doctor in it. The premium reflects the cost-generating behavior of the providers in that particular system. Thus patients may be able to get lower premiums by signing up with economical providers. Economical providers may be able to attract more patients. (Whether they can depends on whether or not patients are offered a choice that includes an alternative delivery system and whether or not they are allowed to keep the savings generated by making an economical choice. See Chapter 5.)

Third, in the insured fee-for-service system, *there are no defined or enrolled populations to whom providers are responsible for giving care.* The responsibility of physicians is limited to those they willingly accept as patients. There is no tangible reward for effective prevention of medical problems or for treating them in less costly ways.

In an alternative delivery system, *the provider organization is responsible for a voluntarily enrolled population.* Thus it can plan the availability of resources to match the needs of this population. Preventing medical problems or treating them in less costly ways is rewarded.

Fourth, in the insured fee-for-service system, *the intermediary pays the bills after the fact.* It does not organize or manage the services. In varying degrees, an alternative delivery system *organizes, provides, or arranges for the services.* Thus it can exercise management controls over both quality and cost and over location, timing, and other aspects of the delivery of services.

The idea of alternative delivery systems is very closely related to the idea of economic competition, which is discussed in Chapter 5. What is important about alternative delivery systems is not the details of their internal organization, but rather what they can do to improve service and reduce cost in a marketplace of competing health care plans. As Walter McClure put it:

> It is not necessary to specify the internal organizational form of the health care plan in order for it to be subject to competitive economic forces. It is only necessary to identify the specific set of providers responsible for delivering health care, so that a premium and benefit package can be established for them. The more flexibility allowed in the organization, the more easily existing professional arrangements can be accommodated in health care plans with minimal modification to establish competitive economic forces. Then consumers will select a far better mix of organizational types than public policy could do. Also, the set of providers in a plan must not include all providers in an area . . . , else there will be no choice and no competition.[3]

But before discussing the desirability of competition, we must learn something about who the competitors are and would be.

EXAMPLES OF ALTERNATIVE DELIVERY SYSTEMS

Prepaid Group Practice

The best-known type of alternative delivery system is the prepaid group practice, of which in 1978 there were about 130 in the United States with a total enrollment of about 6.4 million members.[4] The largest such system is the Kaiser-Permanente Medical Care Program, with about 3.5 million members in seven states in 1978. Other leading prepaid group practices include Ross-Loos in southern California (200,000 members), Group Health Association of Washington, D.C. (109,000 members), Group Health Plan of St. Paul, Minnesota (108,000 members), and Group Health Cooperative of Puget Sound, Seattle, Washington (251,000 members). All but one of these has been in operation for more than thirty years. Two that started around 1970 are Harvard Community Health Plan, Boston (79,000 members), and Georgetown University Community Health Plan, Washington, D.C. (44,000 members).

The essential principles of prepaid group practice are that an organized group of physicians, working together full time, agree to provide comprehensive health care services for a per capita payment, fixed in advance, to a defined population of voluntarily enrolled members. There are many variations on the theme, depending on their origins and sponsorship and the conditions under which they operate. The physicians may be salaried or may receive a per capita payment plus a share of the program's net income. Some prepaid group practice plans own their own hospitals; others do not. Some of the physician groups include a broad range of specialties; others emphasize "primary care" (family doctors, pediatricians, general internists) and refer patients to outside physicians when specialty care is needed. (In such cases the prepaid group practice pays for the specialist's services.) Prepaid group practice plans have been sponsored by industrial companies, labor unions, physician partnerships, consumer cooperatives, insurance companies and Blue Cross, universities, and others.

There is convincing evidence that prepaid group practices are effective in holding the total per capita costs of medical care (premium and out-of-pocket cost) to levels well below those for comparable people cared for under traditional insured fee for service. About fifty studies have been done since 1950 that compare hospital use and total per capita cost of medical care for people within particular employee groups, some of whom have chosen prepaid group practice and some of whom have chosen traditional insurance. The studies are usually adjusted statistically for the effect of different age and sex compositions of the groups being compared. Harold Luft reviewed and analyzed these studies and concluded that the costs in prepaid group practices were some 10 to 40 percent lower.[5] Most of the cost differences could be attributed to hospital-use rates 25 to 45 percent lower than those of groups with traditional insurance. The cost differences cannot be explained away by such factors as differences in age and sex composition or occupation in the groups being compared, previous health status, or government subsidies. (There is an extremely complex pattern of government subsidies, some of which help the fee-for-service sector, some of which help some prepaid groups. The point is not that subsidies do not exist, but that they do not explain away the substantial cost differences.)

One large study compared hospital use by federal employees and their families in the Washington, D.C., area.[6] Some people got their care from the Group Health Association; others, on an insured fee-for-service basis through Blue Cross–Blue Shield. After adjusting for the age and sex composition of the two groups, the study found that the hospital patient days per 1000 persons per year for persons belonging to Group Health were 59 percent of those insured by Blue Cross. Another study compared the costs to Medicare of beneficiaries in six prepaid group practice plans with the costs of a fee-for-service control group, matched for age, sex, and geographic area.[7] The average cost of the former was only 74 percent of the latter. Medicare beneficiaries who regularly get their care from prepaid group practices are free to get the same benefits from fee-for-service providers outside the plan; in this study, the costs of any outside services used were identified and added to the costs of the prepaid group practice beneficiaries.

Some employers are surprised to hear that the *costs* of care are lower in prepaid group practices and other HMOs than in insured fee for service, because the *premiums* are sometimes higher in the HMO. And the premium is the part the employer sees. HMO premiums may be higher because their benefits are more comprehensive and because they do not use coinsurance or deductibles. Coinsurance and deductibles shift the costs to the employees who use medical care. I advise employers that they would be wise to be concerned with *total* cost and not just *premium* cost, for two reasons. First, the trend is for insured benefits to become more comprehensive and for employers to pay an increasing percentage of them. Second, in a competitive labor market the amount the employer will have to pay to attract workers will be increased by higher living costs for employees. Thus in the long run the employer who succeeds in bringing down health care costs in his community, relative to others, will have to pay that much less for labor.

Compared to insured fee for service, the prepaid group model offers many advantages for economy and quality. The method of payment gives the organization a budget set in advance. Its physicians and managers must seek to get the most effective medical care obtainable within that budget. The method of payment also virtually eliminates the administrative burden of billing and collecting from patients or third parties for each service rendered. And an economical division of labor frees the doctors from business management and allows them to concentrate on providing medical care.

Practice in a multispecialty group has advantages independent of the method of payment. These advantages include ease of consultation, which can be a convenience for both the physician and the patient; the "checks and balances" that come from having a patient's treatment considered by physicians from different specialties; and the stimulation and reassurance of mutual professional support. Multispecialty groups keep a single, unified medical record for each patient, which allows each doctor to see what any other physicians are doing to and prescribing for the patient. This can cut down on duplication of costly diagnostic tests, save physician time (since a complete patient history need be taken only once), and provide opportunities for quality control.

As explained in Chapter 3, a major contributor to cost in the fee-for-service sector is excess facilities: underused hospital beds, surgery suites, radiation-therapy units, and the like. The prepaid groups that own their own hospitals have both the ability and the incentive to build or buy only the facilities their enrolled population will need. And they operate less than half the beds per capita as their fee-for-service counterparts. Similarly, the prepaid groups can control the number of physicians, and their specialties, and relate them to the needs of their enrolled members. Prepaid group practices employ relatively more primary-care physicians and fewer surgeons than are in the population as a whole.

Group practices can control the quality of their physicians and have incentives to do so. They can review the qualifications of a doctor before he or she joins and take action to correct poor performance afterward. They can adjust the professional activities of each physician to the tasks that he or she is currently well qualified to perform without threatening the doctor's livelihood. Unlike the fee-for-service sector, in the group-practice setting there need be no financial incentive for a physician to practice beyond his or her competence.

Is the reduction in *cost* achieved at the expense of a reduction in the *quality* of care? "Quality of care" is an extremely complex concept having many dimensions. For reasons explained in Chapter 1, we do not have simple yardsticks to measure it, and such yardsticks are not likely to be developed soon. Although there might well be exceptions in individual cases, I have concluded that in general, the cost reductions have been achieved without sacrificing quality. My reasons for this are the following. First, many educated middle-class consumers, given a choice, often with no difference in cost to themselves, have consistently chosen prepaid group practices and been satisfied with the care received. (Of course, many others have not so chosen.) In fact, my working definition of "good quality care" is "that which is satisfactory to educated middle-class consumers over the long run." As argued in Chapter 3, we should use "consumer-oriented" rather than "provider-oriented" concepts of quality. I say "long run" because I recognize that "you can fool some of the people some of the time. . . ."

Second, various committees, rivals, critics, and others have looked for reductions in quality and have not been able to document them on any systematic basis. Third, when one looks in detail at how the savings are made (the kind of thing discussed in Chapter 3), there is no reason to presume a reduction in quality—quite the contrary. As Harold Luft observed, the main way prepaid groups cut cost is by hospitalizing their members 25 to 45 percent less. It is interesting to observe that as some of the leading fee-for-service multispecialty group practices, such as St. Louis

Park Medical Center in Minnesota and Palo Alto Medical Clinic in California, develop prepaid plans and measure, for the first time, their per capita hospital use, they find that their hospital use looks like that of the prepaid group practices, not like that of the fee-for-service sector in general.[8] The hospital use per capita of local people cared for by the Mayo Clinic also resembles that of the prepaid group practices rather than that typical of the fee-for-service sector. If one accepts as justified the high esteem in which these prestigious groups are held, this finding suggests that the lower amount of hospitalization may be the medically appropriate amount. It also suggests that the essential factor in low hospital use may be related to the multispecialty group-practice style and to the fact that such groups add doctors only as they are needed, and not to the financial incentives in the per capita method of payment.

As a model for reform of the health care system in general, the prepaid group practice has some serious limitations. First, it can take much time and cost to get one started. The experience of the Georgetown University and Harvard Community Health plans and others suggests that several years and several million dollars are required before a new prepaid group practice will reach the financial break-even point. Of course, the start-up time and cost are considerably less when an existing fee-for-service group practice is converted to the prepayment system.

Second, to join a prepaid group practice plan, patients often must change their physicians, something many will be reluctant to do. Thus prepaid groups seem to grow fastest in areas and among population segments characterized by high mobility, where people are required to find new physicians anyway, or where such plans are formed by converting successful fee-for-service group practices to the prepayment mode.

Third, many patients apparently do not prefer this style of care. Some perceive it as impersonal, institutional, or inconvenient. However, we really do not know how many would prefer the prepaid group to the individual-practice style of care, because most Americans have not been given the choice at all and/or on a basis that is geographically accessible and economically fair. Fourth, and even more important, it is evident that this style of practice, although attractive to some physicians, is quite unattractive to many others, who see it as limiting their professional independence too much.[9]

In a national system of fair economic competition, prepaid group practices would be effective competitors. But because of these limitations, they are not likely to dominate the scene. There would be a good deal of room for other kinds of organizations.

Individual Practice Association

The next most common type of alternative delivery system is the individual practice association, or "IPA," sometimes described as a "fee-for-service health maintenance organization." In 1978 there were about seventy IPAs in operation, with about one million members. One of the prototypes was the San Joaquin Foundation for Medical Care, in California. Some say that it was established in 1954 as a way of keeping Kaiser-Permanente out of Stockton. (Although San Joaquin supplied much of the leadership to the IPA movement, its recent role has been primarily that of a traditional third-party claims processor rather than a true alternative delivery system.) Another prototype is the Physicians Association of Clackamas County, Oregon (23,000 members). Among the recent and fast-growing IPAs are Comprecare (33,000 members), in Colorado, and Physicians Health Plan (50,000 members), in Minnesota.

There are many variations on the IPA theme. In fact, the boundary line between the IPA model and the other types of alternative delivery system is often not very clear. The essential principles of the "classical IPA" are these. The physician continues to practice in a private office on a fee-for-service basis. However, as part of the IPA, the physicians agree to provide comprehensive health benefits, including hospital care, lab, and X-ray, to the enrolled membership for a fixed monthly payment. To reconcile fee for service with the fixed payments, the physicians agree to various controls. First, typically, they agree on a maximum fee schedule. When they render a service to a member of the plan, they bill the plan, not the member. Second, they accept "peer review" of the appropriateness of service. This has led individual practice associations to develop a number of cost-control tools, including criteria for patient care such as "model treatment systems" and "preadmission certification." That is, the doctor has to get permission before hospitalizing an IPA member. Third, the association either pays hospital costs or teams up with an insurance carrier that offers a hospital-insurance policy. The premium for the policy reflects the hospital use of those enrolled in the individual practice association. Finally, the physicians accept varying degrees of financial risk. If the money runs low, they may agree to accept a pro rata reduction in fees. In some plans physicians are also liable for costs of inappropriately ordered hospital use or for hospital costs in excess of the budgeted amount.

The individual-practice model offers some substantial advantages. The first is that, compared with a prepaid group practice, an individual practice association can be established more quickly and with a smaller initial investment. It requires a minimal change in the established physician's practice style. Physicians can remain in fee-for-service solo practice and maintain existing doctor-patient and hospital-staff relationships. Patients may be able to enroll in an IPA without changing doctors. Second, fee-for-service practice has positive aspects that should not be overlooked in the present concern with cost. It does reward the doctor for working harder and for being more attractive to patients.

However, despite the apparent ease of start-up, individual practice associations have not grown in number or membership as fast as prepaid group practices have. According to the July 1978 census of health maintenance organizations, only 34 percent of all of the plans representing 14 percent of total membership were IPAs.

IPAs have a credibility problem on the subject of cost reduction. Harold Luft concluded that "there is no evidence that costs for enrollees in individual practice associations are any lower than for people with conventional insurance."[10] Others have looked for such evidence, but their claims have been weakened by the lack of the kind of side-by-side comparison that satisfies the statisticians.[11] I think that the key factor is competition. IPAs have the tools, and they can control costs if they must. For example, the Physicians Health Plan in Minnesota has been able to bring its hospital use reasonably close to that of the other HMOs with which it competes. *Perhaps the most important lesson of the IPA experience is that if economic survival in the face of competition is at stake, physicians will impose on themselves controls they would never dream of accepting if imposed by government.*

Cost control in individual practice associations is weakened by the fact that the physicians are paid on a fee-for-service basis. Thus at the level of the individual decision makers, the financial incentives remain mostly cost-increasing. In a sense the format of the individual practice association assumes that abuse or gross overuse of services by a few doctors is the cause of the cost problem. Peer review curbs the excesses, but it does not do much to motivate a reduction in the costs generated by the majority of doctors whose practices are near the norms.

Individual practice associations like to sign up 75 to 100 percent of the physicians in private practice in their community—many more than the number needed to serve their enrolled members. The main reason is marketing: The association cannot tell prospective enrollees that they will be able to keep their own doctors, unless most of the doctors belong. Another reason is political: to neutralize the opposition of the physicians who oppose alternative delivery systems in principle. But signing up practically all of the doctors means that the association includes the physicians who generate high costs as well as those who are economical. And it means that the association cannot realize the benefits of matching the number and specialty mix of its physicians to the needs of its enrolled population. Thus individual practice associations face a dilemma: One of their main strengths is connected to a serious weakness. I doubt that they will become effective competitors unless they become selective in their physician membership.

Moreover, signing up most of the physicians in an area may look like monopolistic behavior. Whether or not it is depends on whether there are other competing alternative delivery systems in the area whose doctors aren't in the IPA. If there are, the IPA may be a desirable competitive response. If there aren't, monopoly is a problem. The tradition of sponsorship of individual practice associations by county medical societies can make this situation worse. The IPA may then appear to be a device used in restraint of trade for the purpose of fixing prices and blocking competition from other health plans. The use of IPAs in this manner will not be viable in the long run.

Primary Care Network

A third alternative delivery system, best named the "primary care network (PCN)," is based on the primary-care physician (a generalist, or "doctor of first contact," a person who can treat most ordinary medical problems and can direct the patient to the appropriate specialist for the rest). Although there is not an agreed definition, the term usually refers to general and family practitioners, general internists, and pediatricians. The PCN is comparatively new and small. Its largest prototype is the Wisconsin Physicians Service Health Maintenance Program, which was begun at Wild Rose, Wisconsin, in 1970 and covered about 136,000 people in 1978. The SAFECO Life Insurance Company of Seattle started a primary care network in Woodland, California, in 1974. By 1979, SAFECO had enrolled 30,000 members in Washington and California. The Group Health Plan of Northeast Ohio and the Pennsylvania Blue Shield's Comprehensive Health Care Program are based on the same principles. The value of studying them is for the innovative quality of their ideas rather than for the duration and breadth of their experience.

In the SAFECO plan an enrolled member agrees to get all of his care from or through (on referral by) the participating primary-care physician of his choice. No deductible or coinsurance is required. Except for emergencies, services not ordered by the primary-care physician are not covered. A beneficiary who is not satisfied with his doctor may either select another participating physician and remain in the prepaid plan or switch to a conventional insurance plan was coinsurance.

The participating primary-care physician agrees to provide all primary-care services directly and to arrange referrals and to supervise all other care, including specialist services and hospitalization, for each of his or her enrolled beneficiaries. For his or her own services, this physician is paid a negotiated fixed amount per enrolled patient (called a monthly "capitation payment"). The amount depends on the age and sex of the patients, because average medical needs vary with these categories.

An account is also set up for each participating physician from which the bills for all referral services are paid. This account accumulates an amount based on the premiums paid by or for that doctor's patients, less an allowance for the insurance company's costs and less the "capitation payments." The physician must see and approve every bill before it is paid. If there is a surplus in this account at the end of the year, the doctor gets half of it. If there is a deficit, the doctor pays back half of it up to a limit of 5 percent of the capitation payments. (To protect physicians from the unusually high costs of "catastrophic illness," the costs of patients whose annual expenses exceed $5000 are excluded from these calculations and are paid by the insurance company from its reserves.)

A medical director, assisted by a board of participating physicians, monitors use of services, especially hospitalization. Questionable patterns of use are reviewed by a physician advisory board for possible corrective action. The company reports hospital bed-days of about 300 per 1000 per year for employees under age sixty-five and their families, compared with 350 days in Group Health Cooperative of Puget Sound, a prepaid group practice, and 479 for patients with traditional insurance with Blue Cross of Washington State.[12]

As with the other models, there is room for considerable variation on this theme. In the Wisconsin Physicians Service Program, the primary-care physicians are paid on a fee-for-service basis, not capitation. The Wisconsin plan includes specialists; the SAFECO plan is built on primary-care physicians. The Wisconsin plan is sponsored by physicians and endorsed by county medical societies. The SAFECO plan is sponsored by an insurance company. The formulas for sharing in the savings can vary.

I think that this model is particularly important because the existing health insurance industry could use it to transform our national health care economy very quickly. The primary care network can be started with a minimum of both investment and disruption of established practice patterns and relationships among doctors and patients, hospitals, and other doctors. Also, it can be tied into existing group-insurance arrangements. SAFECO's cost to establish its plan in four areas over a four-year period was less than $500,000. The primary care network can start small, with a few doctors and families, and can be extended gradually into a whole system including specialists and hospitals. It can serve small communities. It does not have the large start-up cost of prepaid group practice, and it does not require some 30,000 to 40,000 members to break even. Moreover, it does not require the kind of majority agreement by physicians in the county medical society that has slowed the development of IPAs. An insurer and some primary-care physicians can start a primary care network in a community even if the specialists in oversupply who are threatened by it don't agree.

The primary care network makes the individual primary-care physicians knowledgeable about and accountable for the total health services costs of their enrollees. It gives them an incentive to increase productivity, for example, by employing nurse practitioners. It gives them incentives to emphasize prevention of illness and to instruct patients in self-care. It makes the primary-care physician the "general manager" of the patient's medical care, a much needed role in today's complex health care system.

There are many ways in which the primary care network can cut cost without cutting the quality of care. Primary-care physicians can control their patients' use of hospital services, including length of stay, consultations, duplication of tests, and the like. They can refer patients to appropriate specialists when needed and can choose specialists who are economical in the use of resources. Since the primary-care physician's services are covered by the monthly capitation payment, a great deal of claims processing and bill collecting is eliminated. And the primary care network can inform the participating doctors of prices being charged and can help them to shop wisely. Thus the primary care network creates a market for specialty and hospital services in which the buyers are experts—physicians able to judge quality, need, and appropriateness of services in relation to cost.

The primary care network has many of the advantages of individual practice association without one of its most serious defects. In the IPA the individual doctor is paid fee for service and has no knowledge of or incentive to control total per capita cost of services for his or her enrollees.

Another of the main weaknesses of the classical IPA is that it doesn't do much for the doctor. It offers only restraints, such as maximum fee schedules, controls on use of the hospital, and pro rata reductions in fees. It has been said, with some truth, that "an IPA is merely a defensive alliance against prepaid group practice," and, in fact, a major force sustaining most successful IPAs has been the competitive threat of a prepaid group. The prepaid group practice does offer distinctive advantages to the doctor: a group of professional colleagues, freedom from the chores of managing a small business, regular hours, and stability of income. The primary care network also offers an answer to the question "Why should a successful doctor join one?" In today's professional hierarchy, the specialist commands the most money and prestige. The primary care network makes the family doctor the "general manager of the patient's medical care," thus enlarging his or her role and power within the profession. It allows doctors whose practice style is economical to benefit from that style.

There are potential disadvantages also. Are the incentives to control cost too strong? Will they lead to inadequate service? There might be a problem of preferred-risk selection. A doctor could benefit financially by discouraging high-risk patients from continuing their enrollment with him or her. There might be an economic incentive for a physician to give less than adequate care to patients paid for on a capitation basis, possibly by doing procedures that should have been referred to a specialist. But there are safeguards against such abuses, the most important of which is the dissatisfied patient's freedom to change doctors or health plans. (SAFECO reports that very few patients switch doctors, and the company monitors switches and complaints very carefully.) The design of the incentive formulas can be modified to correct many such problems if they emerge.

And any payment system, including fee for service, must ultimately place a great deal of reliance on the ethics of physicians.

Each of these models is flexible. The variations on each of these themes are many and important. Participating in an organized health plan with built-in cost controls need not be an uncomfortable straitjacket for the physician or the patient. There are enough models to suit the tastes of many—perhaps most. Moreover, I believe that other interesting possibilities would emerge that have not yet done so because we do not have a system of fair economic competition that creates a demand for such innovations.

Altogether, the number of HMOs and similar alternative delivery systems and their memberships have grown rapidly in the 1970s. The number of such plans in operation increased from 52 in 1971 to 203 in 1978. The number increased by 23 percent from 1977 to 1978 alone. Membership increased from about 3.5 million in 1971 to 7.5 million in 1978.[13] It increased 18 percent from 1977 to 1978. This has occurred despite many barriers to HMO growth, described in Chapter 5.

THE SIGNIFICANCE OF ORGANIZED SYSTEMS OF MEDICAL CARE

In the system of independent physicians paid on a fee-for-service basis, community hospitals paid essentially on a cost-reimbursement basis, and patients well insured by third-party intermediaries, none of the actors on the scene has enough control of enough of the variables to be able to create an economical alternative to the costly standard of care that predominates in our country. Each actor must respond within the limits and incentives of this economic framework.

In contrast, an organized system financed on a prepaid or capitation basis can exert substantial influence over the many key variables. An organized system can control the style of care and the accessibility of its services and can, within the limits set by standards of medical care and government regulations, design its program to appeal to one or another type of patient. It might deemphasize hospitalization and apply the savings to improved access to outpatient care. It might allocate more resources to convenient neighborhood primary-care centers and to a more personal style of care, at the expense of less use of specialty care. It might emphasize home care at the expense of high-technology care. It might achieve savings from efficient operations and apply them to broadening its benefits in areas such as preventive care and mental health.

Thus organized systems are not merely devices for financing by capitation the same bundle of services as that offered by insured fee-for-service medicine; nor are they merely incentive schemes for lowering costs or use of services. Rather, they are a framework within which providers can offer very different combinations of services, emphasizing different values, depending on the tastes of the patients served.

A complete program of medical care today requires a large, complex organization. There is need for not only doctors and hospitals, but also a system to guide the patient in their use. For this reason, it makes sense to have a formal organization so that there will be a management responsible for making the parts work well together. The trouble with the solo-practice model of medical care is that the doctor and the hospital jointly provide a service, but nobody has responsibility for overall quality or cost.

Years ago the Defense Department decided to purchase complete airplanes from "prime contractors" rather than buy airframes from one manufacturer and engines from another, only to find they did not fit together. Similarly, as medical care becomes more complex, it will become more important for patients to go to a "prime contractor," an organized system that accepts responsibility for getting the whole job done.

GOOD HMOs, BAD HMOs, AND THE HMO UNDERSERVICE ISSUE

Not all alternative delivery systems, not even federally qualified health maintenance organizations, are good organizations. Just as there are good and bad doctors in the fee-for-service sector, good and bad managers in business and in government, and ethical and unethical people in all walks of life, so too there will be good and bad alternative delivery systems. Some HMOs have been put together on the basis of poor design principles. Some have had poor leadership and have suffered the consequences of some very ill-advised decisions. The fact of being an HMO is definitely not a guarantee of quality or competence.

One point of particular concern is that HMOs may achieve their financial success by underserving their members. The established HMOs, such as Kaiser-Permanente and Group Health Cooperative of Puget Sound, have for many years served such educated middle-class groups as federal and state employees, university faculties, and other teachers. If there were a substantial amount of underservice, one would think that the word would get around and that these people would switch at the next annual enrollment period. I have been unable to find any documented case of a pattern of underservice among such HMOs.

The main basis for the concerns with underservice is the unfortunate experience with the Medicaid-oriented "prepaid health plans" in the early 1970s, mainly in southern California. There, the state government was trying to cut costs in a hurry. It accepted unrealistically low bids for contracts to care for Medicaid beneficiaries from "fly-by-night" enterprises that were created just for the purpose of entering into these contracts. These were not HMOs with established positions in the market. The state also encouraged enrollment practices that interfered with the free choice of the beneficiaries. People were deliberately and systematically misled by false marketing practices. The underservice problem arose from the state government's politically motivated purchasing policies. It did not arise from the nature of HMOs. Many of the doctors who staffed the "Medicaid prepaid health plans" had come from the fee-for-service sector and subsequently returned to it. It would be no more fair to imply that these prepaid health plans were representative of HMOs in general than it would be to imply that the equally scandalous "Medicaid mills" are representative of the fee-for-service sector.

All this is not to say that the financial incentives in the existing HMOs are perfect or that their performance is without shortcomings. We simply do not know what the "right" financial incentives are. There is no logical or empirical basis for determining them *a priori*. And good incentives do not guarantee good performance. Medical care is full of judgment and uncertainty; mistakes are made in any setting, including HMOs.

The most important thing about alternative delivery systems (including HMOs) is that their existence creates the possibility of fair economic competition. And it is through competition that we can find the solutions to the problems of cost, access, and quality of care. If we ensure that every family has a free and fair choice among competing health plans, organizations that make a practice of underserving their members will not last long. The only way to find good methods of organization and good incentives is through experience in a system of fair economic competition among alternative delivery systems.

With competition, some HMOs will fail, just as do businesses in our private-enterprise economy. This is healthy. It drives out the bad ones and keeps the good ones on their toes. It is not a sign that there is something wrong with the HMO idea. I believe that the best guarantee of quality in health care delivery, as in other services, is survival in a fair competitive marketplace. The meaning of such competition, and our experience with it, are discussed in Chapter 5.

5

Economic Competition Among Health Care Financing and Delivery Systems: Principles and Experience

The classical economists, from Adam Smith in 1776 to A. C. Pigou in the 1920s, extolled the virtues of the free-market system. They found that it produces a kind of social optimum in which "the wealth of nations" is maximized. Then the Great Depression of the 1930s produced a wave of disillusionment about the market. Indeed, according to classical theory, a depression could not happen. For the next three decades, the dominant themes in economic thought were criticism of the market and uncritical acceptance of regulation by government as the answer to the failure of the market. The decade following the mid-1960s saw a big increase in government regulation of our economy and social life.

In recent years economists have been reviewing the experience and finding that regulation has its systematic failures also. In an imperfect world, perhaps the market is not the worst alternative. Perhaps its failings can be corrected without resort to what Charles Schultze, Chairman of the

Council of Economic Advisors, has called "the command and control techniques of government bureaucracy."[1] Perhaps we should, to use Schultze's nice phrase, make "public use of private interest" and correct the failings of the market instead of supplanting it with regulation.

This is the great choice we face in the strategy for health care cost control: economic competition or regulation. By "regulation" I mean direct government controls on prices, productive capacity, and the use of services. And by "competition" I mean a market system supported by "procompetitive regulation" designed to help the market achieve society's goals. I am not referring to a return to a completely free market.

This chapter is about competition; Chapter 6, about regulation. This chapter begins with an explanation of the principles of fair economic competition in health care, followed by an explanation of how it is that for the most part, we do not have fair economic competition in health services today. I go on to discuss why we cannot have a completely free market in health services and why some rules are needed if the market is to produce good results. Finally, I review our limited experience with competition and the lessons it can teach us.

PRINCIPLES OF FAIR ECONOMIC COMPETITION

The essential principles of a system of fair economic competition among health care financing and delivery plans are the following.

Multiple Choice

Once a year, each consumer (individual or family) would be offered the opportunity to enroll for the coming year in any one of the health plans operating in his or her area and meeting certain uniform standards governing all health plans. Although traditional insurance plans offering "free choice of doctor" on a fee-for-service basis would be included among the choices, I believe that competition would encourage, and in fact compel, the development of alternative delivery systems with built-in cost controls.

Fixed Dollar Subsidies

The amount of financial help each consumer gets toward the purchase of a health plan membership—from Medicare, Medicaid, an employer, or through the tax laws—would be the same whichever plan he or she chooses. The subsidy might be greater for people with lower incomes than for people with higher incomes, more for the old than for the young, larger for families than for individuals, more for people in one geographic area or bargaining unit than those in another, but not more for people who choose more costly health plans. Thus the financial help each consumer gets would have to be in a fixed dollar amount, independent of his or her choice of health plan. The consumer who chooses a more costly plan would pay the extra cost himself; the consumer who chooses a less costly health plan would save money. Thus the consumer would have a reason to choose wisely, to make a careful judgment as to whether the value offered by a more expensive plan was worth the extra cost.

Same Rules for All Competitors

A uniform set of rules would apply to all health plans. Rules would govern enrollment procedures, premium-setting practices, minimum standards for covered benefits, and information disclosure. The point of such rules would be to ensure that all health plans are competing to provide good-quality comprehensive care at a reasonable cost, not profiting by such practices as selection of preferred risks (see below) or selling deceptive or inadequate coverage.

Doctors in Competing Economic Units

In a system of economic competition, physicians would be organized in competing economic units, such as alternative delivery systems, so that the premium each group charged would reflect its ability to control cost.

CURRENT LACK OF FAIR ECONOMIC COMPETITION IN HEALTH SERVICES

Economic Competition Explained

A frequent response to recommendations that we follow a strategy of economic competition is: "We already have competition in health insurance and health services, and it is not working." This response is based on a lack of understanding of today's system. To be sure, we do see hospitals competing with one another for doctors (who bring in patients) and for prestige, while physicians vie for both patients and professional recognition. And there is vigorous competition in health insurance (that is, insurance carriers compete with one another and with employer self-funded plans for contracts to insure employee groups). But because of the way that health insurance connects to health services, with few exceptions there is no true economic competition in health services. The competition that now exists is not of a kind that rewards economy in the use of resources in either the production or purchase of health care services.

When economists talk about a competitive economy as an efficient way to allocate resources, they are referring to a system in which buyers and sellers are cost-conscious. Each producer pays the full cost of the goods or services he sells. The price at which he sells is set in competition with other sellers. The price he can get is what buyers are willing to pay in view of what other sellers are asking. He cannot raise his price above what other sellers are asking for similar products or services without losing business. His profit margin is the difference between the market price and what it costs him to produce a unit. It is reduced if he lets his production costs increase. So he is cost-conscious in the use of resources.

The consumer has limited resources. If he spends more on one thing, he has less money for other things, so he is motivated to consider the value received for each dollar he spends. The consumer is assumed to be well informed about the price and quality of his purchases before he buys, and his purchases are voluntary. When such cost-conscious buyers and sellers are free to shop around and make the transactions that are of best advantage to themselves, trade produces a kind of social optimum in which all opportunities for mutual gain have been exhausted.

For the most part, these conditions are not satisfied in today's health care economy. For reasons explained in Chapter 2, the insured fee-for-service system does not hold doctors and hospital administrators responsible for the costs they generate. Consumers are not cost-conscious, because their medical purchases are paid for largely by insurance. And consumers are at a large disadvantage when it comes to information about the costs and benefits of various individual health services. If the need is urgent, the consumer's purchase is not well characterized as voluntary.

Most People Don't Have Multiple Choice

Most employed people get their health insurance through their employers. And when the employee is hired, the employer usually presents a single health insurance policy. Several factors appear to have contributed to this practice by employers. First, if one accepts the casualty-insurance model of health care finance, a single insurance policy for the group seems natural. The idea of health care choices has appeal only if there are alternative delivery systems. (A second insured fee-for-service, "free choice of doctor" health plan would not add much to the employee's range of choices.) But until recently, alternative delivery systems didn't exist in most areas. There is a kind of "chicken and egg" problem. The alternatives have a hard time getting started because employers don't offer choices, and employers don't offer choices because alternatives don't exist.

Second, insurers have persuaded employers that they can get a better price for the insurance if they offer a single plan. And some employee benefits managers see a single plan as more comfortable and less work. The trouble with this reasoning is that they are looking only at the administrative costs of health insurance, which are typically a small fraction of the total premium cost. They are assuming, incorrectly, that the health care costs are all for "necessary" care, beyond the control of the insurer.

Third, some union leaders feel that the presence of a single plan makes it easier to keep health benefits under their control. Furthermore, a single health plan for all members is more compatible with labor union philosophy.

But for whatever reason it exists, the practice of offering a single plan creates a major barrier to competition in health services. Alternative delivery systems offering "limited choice of doctor" cannot be an employer's only plan if the employee's freedom of choice of doctor is to be preserved. Thus alternative delivery systems can't get started unless there is acceptance of the "dual-choice" or "multiple-choice" principle.

The Health Maintenance Organization Act of 1973 requires employers to offer their employees the option of joining one group-practice and one individual-practice HMO if such organizations meeting federal standards are operating in their area. This was an important step in the right direction. That such a law was needed shows what a barrier to competition labor-management control of health benefits has become. But it is far from creating the competition we need. HMOs are still too few in number, for the most part too small, and too tightly regulated by the federal and state governments to be able to bring the benefits of competition and choice to most Americans in the foreseeable future. Moreover, the burden is on the HMO to enforce the law by asking the federal government to bring suit against a recalcitrant employer. HMOs are understandably reluctant to antagonize their potential customers. Furthermore, there is much a reluctant employer can do that raises an HMO's costs while technically complying with the law, such as delaying tactics, denying access to employees, or requiring it to print and distribute special brochures.

Employers could adopt the multiple-choice principle and create an effective system of health plan competition. Some already have. But if employers continue to resist the idea, and if we want competition, it will be necessary to change the tax laws either to remove labor-management control of health benefits or to give employers more powerful incentives to offer multiple choice. Also, the definition of the kind of health plan that is allowed to compete needs to be broader than the official definition of a federally qualified HMO.

Employer control of health benefits creates other barriers to health plan competition as well. Even if all employers embraced the principle of multiple choice, the employer-based system of health insurance would add a great deal to the start-up costs of a new alternative delivery system. Before such a health plan can be offered to the employees, it must satisfy the requirements of the employer. About half of the labor force works for employers with fewer than 100 employees. So the new health plan frequently must incur the substantial expense of persuading an employer to offer it as a choice, only to find that it eventually gets five or ten enrollees for its effort. Imagine what your chances of success would be if you started a corner grocery store in an economic system in which you had to make a deal with each person's employer before you could sell groceries to the employee! You would be very likely to spend much of your capital on the costs of making deals with employers and have very little left over to invest in the business. That is what is happening to many health-maintenance organizations trying to get started today.

People whose health care is paid for by government usually don't have choices either. The aged are locked into Medicare, and the eligible poor get Medicaid, both programs based on fee for service and cost reimbursement. For the most part, people do not get a choice of membership in an alternative delivery system.

Most People Don't Get Fixed Dollar Subsidies

Today, Medicare, Medicaid, employers, and tax laws systematically pay more on behalf of beneficiaries who choose more costly health plans or providers. The workings of the tax laws are particularly important.

As explained in Chapter 2, the tax laws motivate employers and employees to agree that the employer pay 100 percent of the health insurance premiums. That way, premiums are paid with employers' pretax dollars instead of employees' after-tax dollars. One consequence of this is that when employees are given choices, the employer will often pay the full premium whichever plan the employee chooses, with the unfortunate result that employees do not have any financial incentive to choose a less costly health plan. For example, in 1978 autoworkers in California had a choice between a Kaiser plan that cost $77 per month and an insured fee-for-service plan that cost $101. The workers who chose Kaiser did not get to keep the savings, because General Motors paid the whole cost either way. Thus many collective-bargaining agreements force the employer to subsidize the employee's choice of a more costly health plan.

My student, Martha Gilmore, did a survey of employer practices in Santa Clara County, California, in 1979. One would expect employers in Santa Clara County to be much more aware of the benefits of competition in health care than employers in most places because the Kaiser program has been active in northern California for more than thirty years and serves more than 1.5 million members there. It would be difficult for a Santa Clara County employer not to have heard of Kaiser. Of a random sample of employers with 500 or more employees, 36 percent offered a single health insurance plan, 42 percent offered a choice but contributed more if the employee chose a more costly plan, and only 22 percent offered both a choice and an equal employer contribution. Among firms with between 25 and 500 employees, 73 percent offered employees a single health insurance plan, 23 percent offered a choice of plan but contributed more on behalf of the employee who took the more costly plan, and only 3 percent offered both a choice and an equal contribution. Of those offering a choice, one-third of the larger employers and three-quarters of the smaller employers paid 100 percent of the premium, whichever plan the employee chose.

This pattern of employer payment of 100 percent of the premium, whichever choice the employee makes, can create a serious barrier to the development of alternative delivery systems. How this happens is illustrated by what was happening in San Mateo County, California, in 1979. Most local government employees there were offered a choice between a traditional insured plan, usually with a premium around $125 per family per month for comprehensive benefits, and membership in the Kaiser program, at about $85 per family per month, with the employer paying the whole premium either way. Two new individual practice associations were trying to enter the market, with family premiums of about $110 per month. Employees who had the more costly insurance had little or no incentive to choose the IPA, at $110, since they could get the same services from the same providers through either their insurance plans or the IPA (actually, with more freedom of choice with insurance), and it was the employer, not the employee, who would save the $15 if the employee joined the IPA.

One of the most important things the new individual practice associations had to offer was cost control. If the employers pay the whole premium, there is no demand (on the part of employees who make the decision) for cost control. What these employers were doing, in effect, was to assure the more costly providers who work in the insured fee-for-service sector that there was no need for them to control costs. (Incidentally, the Health Maintenance Organization Act requires employers to offer only one of these individual practice associations. Unless employers go beyond the minimum requirements of the law, no employees will be given a choice between the two.)

Medicare is based on fee for service and cost reimbursement. Thus it systematically pays more on behalf of people who choose more costly systems of care. (There is a provision for paying health maintenance organizations on a basis meant to reward them for their lower costs, but it is very complex, discriminatory against HMOs and their members, is based on cost reimbursement, and has not been put into operation to any appreciable extent.) For example, in 1970 Medicare paid $202 per capita (on a cost-reimbursement basis) on behalf of beneficiaries cared for by cost-effective Group Health Cooperative of Puget Sound, but paid $356, or 76 percent more, on behalf of similar beneficiaries in the same area who chose to get their care from the fee-for-service sector. On average, for six prepaid group practice plans around the country included in the study from which these data came, Medicare paid 36 percent more on behalf of similar beneficiaries who chose fee for service.[2] And it is in the nature of Medicare cost reimbursement that this subsidy to the fee-for-service sector will increase as the cost differential widens. Medicare beneficiaries could get their care from the less costly provider, but they were not allowed to keep for themselves most of the savings generated by that choice, in either lower premiums or better benefits. The government kept the savings generated by their decisions. It simply is not fair competition if the government systematically pays more on behalf of similar people who enroll with one type of competitor than with another.

From the point of view of those who are eligible, Medicaid pays the entire cost of covered benefits. But again, most Medicaid providers are paid on a fee-for-service and cost-reimbursement basis. Medicaid usually has limits on fees for individual services. But providers can increase their Medicaid revenues by prescribing a greater volume of services for the same medical condition. Thus Medicaid also pays more on behalf of people who choose more costly providers.

It should not be at all surprising that the alternative delivery systems with built-in cost controls have grown slowly, when one considers that such large powers as the United States government and the auto industry, not to mention the local government agencies of San Mateo County, in effect pay large subsidies to the fee-for-service sector on behalf of people who choose not to enroll in the less costly systems of care.

Different Rules for Different Competitors

Equal rules are not applied to all competitors now. The various competitors are regulated by different levels of government in different ways. Federally qualified HMOs are regulated by the Department of Health and Human Services and by states. Health insurance is regulated by state insurance commissioners. HMOs must practice "community rating"; for the most part, insurers are free to "experience rate" (see below). HMOs must offer a comprehensive package of benefits with very limited copayments and no deductibles; insurers are free to cover fewer benefits and to use any amount of coinsurance and deductibles. In effect, HMOs are required to provide necessary services without limit, whereas insurers can, and generally do, limit the amount they will pay on behalf of someone with a major illness. Of course, in doing this, the insurers are acting as agents for employers. The point is that we are far from applying equal rules to all health care financing and delivery systems.

Most Doctors Are Not in Competing Economic Units

As explained in Chapter 2, health care financing is dominated by "free-choice-of-doctor" insurance plans. The medical profession has traditionally insisted on this principle. Also as explained in Chapter 2, the effect is to rule out economic competition among providers. The well-insured consumer has no compelling reason to care what costs his or her doctor generates. As well as "free choice of doctor," consumers should have "free choice of alternative delivery system" and financial responsibility for the choice.

WHY WE CANNOT HAVE A COMPLETELY FREE MARKET IN HEALTH INSURANCE

I believe that fair economic competition of alternative delivery systems would produce desirable results. It would force the health services industry to be more responsive to the desires of consumers. Health care organizations that did a good job of satisfying their customers—including controlling costs—would survive and prosper. Health plans that did a poor job would lose customers and risk being driven out of business. Thus in the long run the surviving plans would be the ones that offered a good value to their customers. Consumers and providers would be able to benefit by joining health plans that use resources wisely. The health care financing and delivery system would be transformed gradually and voluntarily, by millions of people, each seeking what is in his or her own best interest, from today's system with cost-increasing incentives to one with built-in incentives for consumer satisfaction and cost control.

But although I recommend that employers and government direct their efforts toward the creation of such a market system, I do not recommend a return to a completely free market in health insurance. I take it as given that we want affordable health insurance to be available to every person in the United States. And the desirable competition I am referring to would be focused on the quality, accessibility, and economy of care and not, for example, on the ability of health insurers to select only healthy people to insure. If we want to achieve these goals, we must have rules to channel the competition along socially desirable lines.

There are four basic reasons why we cannot have a completely free market in health insurance. Reflection on them should help us to understand better the rules that are needed to make a private competitive market system work well in serving society's needs.

"Free Riders"

Clearly we cannot have a system in which people are allowed not to buy health insurance until they get sick. People could take advantage of such a system. They could go without paying premiums until they got sick and then buy insurance. The premium then would necessarily be equal to the expected cost of their care (plus administrative costs). There would be no "insurance" in the sense of spreading the risk of illness. The well would pay no premiums; the sick would bear the full cost of their care.

On the other hand, we really cannot have a system in which we say to people, "If you didn't insure when you were well, we won't let you insure when you are sick." As a society, we won't let people suffer seriously or die for lack of medical care. We do, and will continue to, provide a "safety net," and so we have to pay for that net. Therefore, we must have what amounts to compulsory premium contributions, and this comes about through some form of tax. We can, and often do, give this some nicer sounding name such as "employer-mandated premium contributions" or "earnings-based premiums" or "refundable tax credits," but these all amount to compulsory insurance-premium contributions by one or another form of tax. And we do provide substantial taxpayer support for health insurance through Medicare, Medicaid, and the exclusion of employer-provided health benefits from an employee's taxable income, as described in Chapter 2.

Recall from Chapter 1 that people have a great deal of control over the timing of their medical care. I gave an example there of a family that found four of its children in need of open-heart surgery and switched at the next annual enrollment from a low-cost health insurance plan to an HMO with comprehensive prepaid benefits in order to get all the heart surgery paid for. This is an example of the kind of thing that does and would happen if people were allowed an annual choice between an insurance plan with high deductibles and coinsurance and a low premium, and a comprehensive plan without coinsurance or deductibles such as those usually offered by health maintenance organizations. A family could buy the plan with the low premiums until one of its members developed a chronic condition or until it had accumulated substantial medical needs. The family could switch to the comprehensive plan for a year, get these services fully paid by insurance, and then switch back to the insurance plan with the low premiums.

This is not merely a hypothetical problem. It is a significant problem in the real world. Even a highly efficient, effective health maintenance organization could not survive in competition with a "catastrophic expense only" plan and annual open enrollment. What the HMO would in effect be doing in such a case would be granting a free option to join it within twelve months or less—six months on average. Such an option would have a real and substantial value, and the HMO would have to be allowed to charge for it.

Thus a workable competitive market system depends on limiting people's choices or some other device to prevent people from taking advantage of the system. One such device is a lower limit on the cost of the insurance plans and alternative delivery systems that are allowed to compete. For example, in the Federal Employees' Health Benefits Program, described later in this chapter, the federal government, as employer, contributes 60 percent of the average premium of six of the largest health plans in its multiple-choice system. There would be no point in a federal employee's choosing, or a health plan's offering, a policy with a premium less than the government's contribution. For an employee to make such a choice would be, in effect, to throw money away. This contribution formula effectively limits the range of choice. Another such device could be a charge for the option of switching to the comprehensive plan, a "retainer fee" paid by the "catastrophic expense only" subscribers to the comprehensive plans equal to the actuarial value of the option. (Today, HMOs generally compete in employee groups for whom the alternative is fairly comprehensive insurance.)

Preferred-Risk Selection

In a completely free market situation, health insurers would prosper by skillfully classifying people according to their expected medical costs and then winning the business of healthy people by offering to insure them for low premiums. Insurers who charged healthy people higher premiums in order to subsidize the costs of other people more likely to be sick would lose the business of the healthy people. Thus in the extreme the free competition of insurers would eventually result in each person's being charged a premium essentially equal to the expected costs of his or her own medical care.

Experience rating of groups by insurers is a form of this at the group level. Recall that experience rating means that the premium for each group is based on its own medical-expense experience, not on that of the community as a whole. I believe that experience rating violates one of the principles on which health insurance should be based—that the well should help pay for the medical care of the sick. Without this principle, health insurance for people with high medical risks would be unaffordable. (This principle is based on the view that sickness is largely an involuntary misfortune and that the sick are already burdened by their illness and should not be required to pay for extensive care entirely with their own money. Of course, in reality sickness is a complex mixture of misfortune and self-inflicted ill health. If we had a practical way of sorting this out, there would be a case for making people pay for their self-inflicted illnesses but not for misfortunes. Although such ideas, including rewards for healthful lifestyles, are attractive in theory, the range of their practical application is quite limited.)

In a workable system of fair competition intended to make affordable health insurance available to all, we must require all insurers (or at least all those whose policies are eligible for tax subsidies) to accept the bad risks (those who need the insurance most) along with the good risks and to charge them the same premium. The usual terms for this are "periodic open enrollment" and "community rating" of premiums. "Open enrollment" in this case means open to all citizens or eligible persons in the system. "Community rating" means charging the same premium for the same benefits to all persons in the community. In Chapter 7 I propose a modified system of community rating called "community rating by actuarial category." The idea is to require insurers to charge the same premiums for the same benefits to all persons in the same demographic category, such as "adults aged forty-five to sixty-five," but to allow higher premiums to be charged to people in categories with higher average medical costs. Insurance is still made affordable for people in the higher-cost categories by providing them with higher government subsidies. In this way the well help to pay for the cost of care of the sick through the tax system as well as through the health insurance system.

Income Distribution

Most Americans consider access to a decent level of medical care to be a part of the right to "life, liberty, and the pursuit of happiness." Thus we are not willing to leave the distribution of medical purchasing power to the market and other forces that determine income distribution. In programs such as Medicare, Medicaid, and tax-supported county hospitals, we have shown that we accept subsidies of purchases of medical care for low-income people. But this does not mean that the government must itself be the purchaser of medical care for the poor. Indeed, the record of government as the purchaser or provider of such services is not very good. A more efficient and effective way to subsidize medical care for the poor can be through both a system of "income-related premium subsidies" that are large enough to enable them to purchase membership in a good-quality comprehensive health care plan and a multiple choice of the competing private health plans that serve their area.

Information Cost

For a competitive market to produce a socially desirable result, it is necessary that buyers be reasonably well informed about the alternatives they are considering and be able to make intelligent choices for themselves. (Not "all the buyers all of the time," but at least "most of the buyers most of the time.") The effective working of a competitive market system can be impaired if it is too costly for buyers to become well informed. Health care and health insurance are extraordinarily complex fields, poorly understood even by the experts. Insurance policies are often very complex because insurers rely on complicated limitations and exclusions to control their costs and because some insurers seek to avoid price competition by making their policies difficult to compare with others. For this market to work well, I believe that there must be a systematic program by employers and government to make it easy for consumers to understand and compare alternative health plans.

One important part of such a program would be standardization of the list of covered services so that consumers can compare health plans without having to master many pages of fine print or to make actuarial comparisons of one complex package with another. To make price comparisons easy, we must require all health plans to quote premiums for at least one standard package of covered services. We also need a certain amount of information disclosure comparable to that required of publicly held companies by the securities laws, so that people can make informed judgments about the services for which they are contracting.

To summarize, for a workable competitive private-market system that makes affordable health insurance available to everybody, we need some form of mandatory premium contributions or what amounts to the same thing, substantial tax subsidy; some limits on the range of choices so that people cannot take advantage of the system in ways that undermine it; periodic open enrollment; community rating; common basic benefits in all plans; subsidies of health plan membership purchases by low-income people; standardization of benefit packages and other aspects of policies; and information disclosure.

EXPERIENCE WITH HEALTH PLAN COMPETITION

Fair economic competition among alternative health care delivery systems and health insurance plans is not merely a set of theoretical principles, a collection of untried notions of untested practicality. It is not a concept to which we can respond only at an abstract and speculative level. On the contrary, it is a demonstrated practical fact. Some large employee groups have had fair multiple choice for years. And a few communities have effective health plan competition. Indeed, my understanding of the principles explained above was derived from observation of these examples. Each of these cases illustrates some important points about the likely results of competition. I recommend that people who have questions or doubts about the feasibility or effectiveness of competition attempt to resolve them by looking at these experiences.

The Federal Employees' Health Benefits Program (FEHBP)

The Federal Employees Health Benefits' Program (FEHBP) went into operation in 1960 and by 1978 was providing health insurance for about 10 million employees, retirees, and their dependents. Each beneficiary is offered an annual multiple choice of private health plans, including a governmentwide "service benefit plan" (Blue Cross–Blue Shield), a governmentwide "indemnity benefit plan" (Aetna Life and Casualty), each with a "high option" and a "low option," twelve "employee organization plans" tailored to the special needs of particular groups such as foreign service personnel, and more than seventy "comprehensive plans," which are mostly individual-practice associations and prepaid group practices. Because the "comprehensive plans" are local in nature, they are not all available to all federal employees. The available number of them in any area may range from zero in many places to three or four in the best-supplied areas.

The government, as employer, contributes a fixed amount on behalf of each employee equal to 60 percent of the average premium of six of the largest plans. (The government contribution cannot exceed 75 percent of any particular premium. Therefore, it pays somewhat less in the case of some of the "low-option" plans.) The contribution was about $25 per month for an individual and $60 per month for a family in 1979. The employee pays the rest. Thus the employee has a choice and a financial incentive to consider the cost when making that choice.

The program works with remarkable simplicity. The government does not regulate the prices charged by the health plans or by the providers, and it does not get into the complexities of cash-flow management or claims administration that burden many employers. The administrative expense of the Office of Personnel Management, the managing agency, is less than a quarter of one percent of the revenue. William Hsiao, an actuary at the Harvard School of Public Health, did a comparison of the costs of claims administration under Medicare and under the FEHBP.[3] He found that the average cost to process a claim was 26 percent higher in Medicare than in the Federal Employees program, after dissimilar functions were eliminated from the comparison.

A comparison of the laws and regulations governing the FEHBP and Medicare illustrates the simplicity of the former. The law creating the FEHBP is 8 pages long; the Medicare law is 142 pages long (Titles XI and XVIII of the Social Security Act). The FEHBP regulations are 16 pages long; the Medicare regulations fill 400 pages. At the next level down in the pyramid of paperwork are instructions to participants in each program. Medicare's Health Insurance Manuals contain more than 10,700 pages! More than 2700 revisions have been issued since the program started in 1966. Information, instructions, and forms published by the Office of Personnel Management for the FEHBP come to fewer than 100 pages.

I believe that this shows that the principles on which Medicare is based are extremely complex, indeed unworkable in practice. On the other hand, in the FEHBP we have a large-scale example, in operation over a long period of time, that shows that the principles of fair economic competition are very simple and practical.

I have heard many arguments against multiple choice and economic competition in health insurance: "Consumers aren't capable of making such choices"; "Multiple choice of health plan would be very costly to administer"; "They'll all take the cheapest plan, and quality will be sacrificed." The experience of the FEHBP shows that these, and most of the other, arguments against such competition are not supported by experience.

In a history of the Federal Employees program presented in 1964, Andrew Ruddock of the Civil Service Commission brought out both its effectiveness and its potential as a model on which many groups can agree.

> The program finally authorized by Congress permits a wide range of choice of plans by all employees and was, in effect, a negotiated compromise

among many divergent and highly organized interests. It was the only approach which at any time during the legislative process gained acceptance by all of the principals: the American Medical Association, Blue Cross–Blue Shield, insurance companies, employee unions, group and individual practice prepayment plans, and the Federal Government as the employer. Although there can be no doubt that the "single plan" approach would have been most desirable from the standpoint of administrative simplicity, now that we have learned to live with the administrative problems which stem from multiple choice, it becomes equally clear that the wide choice of plans has produced a program which is more effective in meeting the needs of Federal employees and their dependents. . . . It was anticipated by many that serious administrative problems would develop that would require continual legislation of a perfecting and remedial nature. This has not been the case.[4]

Some people ask me: "If the FEHBP is such a good idea, why hasn't it transformed the health care economy and brought costs under control?" My answer is that it *has* helped, but that fortunately for the taxpayers, federal employees remain a small percentage of the population. For the principles of fair economic competition to have a chance to transform the health care system, they must be applied to a majority of the population in a community. Figuratively speaking, this takes us to Hawaii.

Hawaii

In Hawaii more than 80 percent of the working population and about 72 percent of the total civilian population receives its medical care through one of two competing health plans. Thus the two health plans together are large enough to have a decisive impact on the total delivery system.

The larger of the two plans—Hawaii Medical Service Association (HMSA)—is a not-for-profit community-service organization and uses the fee-for-service mode of payment typical of Blue Shield plans. But it has developed cost controls that are much more effective than those used elsewhere by third-party intermediaries. The physician fees HMSA will pay are not allowed to increase faster than inflation. HMSA has also worked to control hospital charges and the amount of hospital use. In 1977 HMSA's fee-for-service plan covered about 484,000 people, about 57 percent of the state's civilian population.[5]

In 1972 HMSA also inaugurated the Community Health Program, in which the care is provided by nine physician groups that are paid on a per capita, as opposed to a fee-for-service, basis. By 1977 this program covered about 23,000 people.

The other large plan is the Kaiser-Permanente program, which entered Hawaii in 1958. By 1977, it had about 107,000 enrolled members, representing 13 percent of the state's civilian population and 16 percent of the population on Oahu, where Kaiser's main facilities are located.

There is little question but that the two plans compete vigorously. More than 50,000 federal, state, and local government employees, including the University of Hawaii, are offered a choice of plan and a fixed employer contribution toward the plan of their choice. Most private-sector employers still do not apply the principles of fair economic competition to health care. In 1975 only about one-quarter of all the private-sector employees in the state were offered a choice; for about 60 percent, the employer paid the full premium for the employee's coverage. The combination of dual choice and an equal fixed-dollar contribution applied to only a few percent of private-sector employees. Nevertheless, competition has been effective in enough of the market to make its results very beneficial to all consumers and employers.

Kaiser's entry into the market put pressure on HMSA to improve its benefit coverage and to strengthen its cost controls. Kaiser, in turn, found it necessary to depart from its traditional style of delivering all of its services in large medical centers and to set up five small outpatient clinics on Oahu at locations convenient to members, in order to compete effectively with HMSA's individual-practice style. Kaiser and HMSA both report hospital use for employees and their families (that is, the under sixty-five age group) at or below 400 days per 1000 per year. Even after adjusting for the age of the population, Hawaii's hospital use is about 75 percent of the national average. Hawaii has about 3 short-term community hospital beds per 1000 civilian population, compared with a national average of about 4.6. Thus the excess of hospital beds that adds so much to costs in most areas is not a problem in Hawaii. As a result, hospital cost per capita through the 1970s was about two-thirds of the national average, despite the fact that the cost of living generally was about 20 percent above the national average. HMSA and Kaiser premiums for comprehensive care are among the lowest in the Federal Employees Health Benefits Program.

Various factors besides competition contribute to this desirable situation in Hawaii. The population is young. Cultural factors and healthful lifestyles play a part. But based on direct observation as well as study of the data, I believe that vigorous and effective competition between HMSA and Kaiser has been the key factor in achieving these lower costs. Both organizations make strenuous efforts to hold down costs while giving good service and comprehensive benefits to their members, in order to remain competitive with each other. And the fact that the two competitors dominate the market is important, because individual providers have a hard time escaping the cost controls of one or the other health plan.

Minneapolis–St. Paul

In November 1978 *Fortune* writer Edmund Faltermayer reported: "In the Twin Cities, competition in medical care has arrived. Aggressive health maintenance organizations are holding price increases to a single digit, and customers love the product."[6] What has happened? And how did it come about?

The Twin Cities' experience with seven competing health maintenance organizations is apparently the result of three forces: some pioneering HMOs which started a "domino effect," enlightened employers who decided to offer their employees a choice of HMOs and to make it easy for HMOs to get started, and Dr. Paul Ellwood, who conceived the market-oriented "health-maintenance strategy" and sold it to the employers.

The Twin Cities' experience illustrates several important points about health plan competition. One is the decisive role of employers. If enough employers in a community adopt the principles of economic competition and help alternative delivery systems to get started, they can trigger a "self-sustaining chain reaction" of competition.

Also illustrated is the variety of origins of HMOs and reasons people have for starting them. The first HMO in the Twin Cities was Group Health Plan, a consumer cooperative started in 1957. By 1970, it served about 36,000 members. The second was started in 1972 by the St. Louis Park Medical Center, a leading multispecialty group practice in a Minneapolis suburb. The leaders of St. Louis Park recognized several key factors about their practice. First, because referrals to their specialists were declining as more specialists set up practice in Minnesota, they felt a need for some organized effort to secure future referrals. Second, they recognized their own efficiency and their own conservative use of hospitalization. As a part of the traditional insured system, the benefit of these efficiencies was spread among policyholders in general. By creating their own health care financing plan, they could realize the benefit for themselves and their enrolled members. Third, they were attracted by the simplicity of the capitation financing system. It would mean a substantial reduction in paperwork through elimination of billing and collection for individual services to enrolled members. Moreover, as medical leaders, they were persuaded that competition of alternative delivery systems was a logical way to improve the performance of the health care system. By the summer of 1979, they had enrolled 60,000 members, compared with Group Health Plan's 131,000.

Following St. Louis Park, five other HMOs entered the market. The Ramsey Health Plan, based at the St. Paul Ramsey Hospital, was started in 1972 to care for Ramsey County employees, but was subsequently opened to other groups. SHARE Health Plan, started as a mutual-benefit association for railroad employees, was reorganized and opened to other groups in 1974. The Nicollet-Eitel Health Plan started in 1973 as a joint venture between the Nicollet Clinic, a multispecialty group practice, and Eitel Hospital. In 1974 Blue Cross–Blue Shield sponsored "HMO in Minnesota," a financial and marketing organization that contracts with independent physician groups to care for its enrolled members on a per capita payment basis. And finally, in 1976 the Hennepin County Medical Society created the Physicians Health Plan, an individual practice association with more than 1200 participating doctors, as a competitive response to the others.

Employers in the Twin Cities took an active interest. In 1972 eighteen companies contributed $40,000 each to form the Twin Cities Health Care Development Project, which helped new HMOs to get started. In addition to educating other employers about the advantages of HMOs, it sought to create a legislative climate that would be sympathetic to HMOs. In 1976 it was reorganized as the National Association of Employers on Health Maintenance Organizations. The most important thing the employers did was to offer the HMOs to their employees and to present them from a positive point of view. Many offered multiple choice and a fixed dollar contribution. They invited HMOs to make presentations to employees on company time and aided in the distribution of informative materials.

This understanding and support by employers was of decisive importance, and the results have been impressive. HMO membership grew from 36,000 in 1970 to more than 300,000 by 1979. Over most of the decade, total HMO membership grew 28 percent per year. By 1979, it reached 16 percent of the population in the metropolitan area and higher percentages in some employee groups. For example, 65 percent of General Mills's employees in the Twin Cities area had enrolled in an HMO, as had 65 percent of Cargill's, 44 percent of Honeywell's and 36 percent of Control Data's. (On the other hand, about 4 percent of the 3M Company's employees had chosen HMOs, reflecting in part that company's lack of support for the idea.)

Some employers have criticized the idea of multiple choice of health plan on the grounds that it requires more administrative effort. The experience of the Twin Cities employers does not support this contention. Control Data offers five plans; Honeywell, six. Control Data's management has told me that the costs are small compared with the benefits. This has also been the experience of other employers who offer multiple choice. The experience also shows that employees can cope with five or six choices; they are not bewildered by them, as some critics of competition have predicted. (Of course, of six or seven HMOs in the metropolitan area, no more than two or three are likely to have locations convenient to any particular consumer.)

The results of this competition have been lower costs and better service for those who have joined HMOs. Under competitive pressures, the HMOs started placing clinics in locations convenient to members and lengthening their hours of operation. From 1974 to 1978, St. Louis Park Medical Center increased its primary-care clinics from five to seventeen locations. Written complaints have been few, and consumer satisfaction appears to be high. Satisfactory cost comparisons are hard to make because of the many variables involved, but a key indicator is hospital days per

1000 enrollees per year. Jon Christianson and Walter McClure of Inter-Study report that the HMOs average about 500 days for their members, compared with about 850 days for similar people (in Minneapolis and nationally) on traditional insurance.[7] From 1974 to 1977, aggregate HMO premiums increased 18 percent per year versus 21 percent for Blue Cross–Blue Shield for Minnesota state employees. The two largest HMOs—Group Health and Med Center—increased their family premiums 13 and 14 percent per year, respectively. (Initially, HMO premiums are usually higher than insurance premiums because their benefits are more comprehensive and they do not use substantial copayments or deductibles. But gradually, in the Twin Cities market the HMO premiums are falling below the insurance premium rates.) InterStudy reports that hospital expenditures per capita in the Twin Cities grew an average of 9.8 percent per year in 1977 and 1978, compared with a national average increase of 13.4 percent.[8]

It is still too early to tell how much of an impact the HMOs will have on aggregate per capita costs in the Twin Cities, because HMO membership still accounts for only one-sixth of the population. A substantial part of what we have seen so far may simply be the effect of the more cost-conscious physicians selecting themselves out of the insured fee-for-service system. For example, the doctors at the St. Louis Park Medical Center apparently have not changed their hospital-use practices. The real cost reductions will come when the growth of HMOs forces a better matching of numbers of doctors and hospital beds to the needs of the population. That will require the closing or shrinking of hospitals and, perhaps, the retirement or relocation of some of the more costly physicians. That had not happened to any appreciable extent by 1979.

People dismiss Hawaii as an example of what competition can do for American health care in general on the grounds that it is not representative of most areas. Although every metropolitan area has its own special characteristics, Minneapolis–St. Paul is harder to dismiss on these grounds.

Project Health, Multnomah County, Oregon

These examples of health plan competition all serve the employed middle class. What about the poor?

The poor have special problems with respect to health care. They are more likely than other people to have health problems. They are difficult to place with health care organizations that serve middle-income people unless either some mechanism is devised to subsidize the extra costs of their care or some way is found to ensure that all health plans take a fair share of high-risk people, including the poor. There is a great deal of fluctuation in the incomes of poor people in some categories. If their eligibility for medical assistance depends on income, these fluctuations may be translated into fluctuations in health plan membership, with breaks in the continuity of care and wasteful administrative costs. Some of the unemployed poor will be less likely than employed people to be able to understand health plan alternatives. And coinsurance and deductibles, because of their cost, are more likely to serve as barriers to needed care for low-income people. Thus comprehensive prepaid plans seem particularly appropriate for low-income people. Can people with these needs be served by a competitive market of health care plans? Project Health of Multnomah County, Oregon, has shown that they can be.

In 1973 Multnomah County sold the hospital that it operated as "the provider of last resort" for the medically indigent and created a new county agency, Project Health, which serves as broker, counselor, and advocate for the poor rather than as provider of care. It contracts with six comprehensive prepaid health plans on a per capita basis. (Three are health maintenance organizations that serve the community in general. One is a university medical center.) Eligible persons are offered their choice from among these plans. Project Health pays the full premium to the health plan and charges each enrolled family a fee (usually comparatively small) based on the family's income and choice of plan.

The family that chooses a more costly health plan pays more. However, these low-income families are not required to pay the whole difference. If they were, the more expensive health plans would be out of reach, and low-income people would be concentrated in the least costly plan. One of Project Health's objectives in seeking "mainstream care" is to avoid concentrating low-income people in one health plan or facility, and the fees were set with a view to distributing the clients evenly over the various health plans.

More important, a family whose income increases does not lose its health plan membership, as can happen under Medicaid. Instead, its monthly contribution increases. Thus Project Health was responsive to the special needs of the poor in the context of a "mainstream" multiple-choice competitive market system.

Some people have told me that the competitive market system cannot work in health care to serve the poor. The experience of Multnomah County shows that they are wrong. However, the principles of fair economic competition have to be adapted to the special needs of the poor. And reform of the system that serves the middle class is a prerequisite for achieving "mainstream care" for the poor on an affordable basis. Project Health was possible because of the existence of HMOs serving the employed people in Multnomah County.

WHAT CAN WE EXPECT FROM THE FAIR ECONOMIC COMPETITION OF ALTERNATIVE DELIVERY SYSTEMS?

What is the likely outcome of the competition of alternative delivery systems? If these have been the actual results of competition in rather limited situations and adverse circumstances, what could we realistically expect if fair economic competition became the norm? Would it really solve the problem of health care costs? I believe that the answer is yes, but the solution would not come quickly.

We should not expect a great deal from partial efforts where competition of alternative delivery systems affects only a small part of a community. In fact, the establishment of an efficient alternative delivery system may even evoke perverse economic responses from the insured fee-for-service sector. Suppose that a prepaid group practice is established in a community and that it cares for its enrolled members with half of the number of doctors and hospital beds per capita as are used by the insured fee-for-service sector. As the prepaid group practice grows in membership, the first result will be more doctors and more beds per capita serving the majority of the community that remains with insured fee for service. For reasons explained in Chapter 2, this will mean higher, not lower, costs per capita in the fee-for-service sector.

The insured fee-for-service sector is not tightly organized like a single firm, and it does not exhibit normal competitive economic responses. Established providers will not cut costs in an effort to retain customers. They will merely raise prices to offset the reduced volume of business and pass them on to the third-party payors. If many employers and the government are willing to pay the full cost of health insurance for those who choose the more costly fee-for-service sector, this process could go on forever. Indeed, it is remarkable how little competitive economic response has been stimulated in the fee-for-service sector in California by the large and fast-growing Kaiser-Permanente program there. I attribute this lack of response to the fact that for the most part, employers and government have not forced the fee-for-service sector to compete on a fair economic basis. This should temper our optimism about what one HMO can do to stimulate reform in the fee-for-service sector.

The potential competitive impact of HMOs in a market dominated by insured fee for service may also be attenuated by other factors. The HMO must compete for doctors and for members. The pay the HMO must offer will be influenced by what doctors can earn in the insured fee-for-service sector, in which the normal economic restraints do not apply. As service improves for the consumers served by the fee-for-service sector (because of its higher doctor-population ratio), the HMO will be inhibited from cutting cost further if that means less convenience or accessibility for members. The fee-for-service sector sets the community standards of care (such as the appropriate number of diagnostic tests for a particular problem or the number of days in the hospital after a heart attack), which may be very costly. But the HMO will need to adhere to them to attract members and to limit its vulnerability to malpractice claims. Moreover, if the HMO uses beds in community hospitals rather than operating its own hospitals, it may be forced to bear part of the cost of the excess beds.

The financial incentives for a not-for-profit HMO to grow will be much weaker than those for a for-profit industrial company for which increased size would mean greater economies of scale and experience and improved profitability. Most HMOs are not-for-profit entities, which means that they will have relatively weak financial incentives to press their cost advantage and to grow as quickly as they can. Some HMOs are consumer cooperatives, run by and for their present members. In some cases the members, acting in their own short-run best interest, have been reluctant to vote dues high enough to generate the capital required for expansion.

All of these factors should help us to recognize that bringing the benefits of competition to most people won't be easy. It won't come as the automatic consequence of a few simple actions. Employers and government will have to make a sustained effort to make it happen. The creation of competition will require that most people in each community be offered fair multiple choice and that physicians, business, and other institutions take the lead in establishing alternative delivery systems.

Even if fair multiple choice is offered to most people and alternative delivery systems are established, the benefits will not come overnight. It takes time to develop alternative delivery systems. However, I do believe that many established health insurers could convert their business from the third-party reimbursement model to the primary care network fairly quickly. People value their established relationships with their physicians, and they will change them only slowly and usually not for a small difference in price. Doctors and patients are understandably wary of new organizational schemes. They will want to see how each innovation works before they can be confident that it is a change for the better. The health services industry is based on many institutions with long traditions and deep roots in their communities. Many people will change their health plans only reluctantly and slowly.

There are no easy routes to health services reorganization. It will take time and a great deal of effort by many people in many localities. What I am proposing here is fundamental, long-term reform of the health care delivery system, not just another "quick fix."

But delivery-system reform would happen if most people were given fair multiple choice. The economic advantage of the efficient organized systems is too great for them not to win out if given a fair chance to compete. And the reform would happen much more quickly and more effectively if employers and government would work together to ensure that every consumer had a choice of all of the alternative delivery systems meeting reasonable standards operating in his or her area. The growth of new alternative delivery systems is slowed a great deal by the fact that they must first persuade and make a deal with the employer of each potential customer before they can sell their program to the customer. The cost of overcoming such artificial barriers could be greatly reduced if employers and government took appropriate steps.

If fair multiple choice became the rule and alternative delivery systems were established in each community, I believe that we would see competition not just in price, but also in all aspects of health care delivery. As we have seen in Hawaii and the Twin Cities, the alternative delivery systems would compete in quality, accessibility, and content of care. If the consumers want more convenient access to care, the competing delivery systems will provide it. If the consumers want more emphasis on health-maintenance service and prevention of disease, the competing delivery systems will provide that also.

But competition on the basis of price would also be important. Consumers would be cost-conscious in their choice of health plan because under the rules of fair economic competition, those who choose a more costly system of care would pay the full extra cost themselves in the form of higher premiums. Consumers would not be willing to pay higher premiums unless they saw extra value. As we saw in Chapter 4, Harold Luft found that prepaid group practices cared for their enrolled members for a total cost (premium and out of pocket) 10 to 40 percent less than the costs of care of similar people under insured fee for service. I think that 25 percent is a good representative average figure. And these cost reductions have been achieved in the absence of economic competition from other alternative delivery systems. Because many employers and government pay the full costs of health insurance, these cost reductions were achieved in an economic environment in which many of the customers had little or no reason to be cost-conscious. I am confident that more cost reduction could be achieved if it were a matter of competitive necessity—that is, if the customers were demanding it.

SAFECO reports that its primary care network in Seattle competes effectively with one of the best prepaid group practices. And Hawaii Medical Service Association competes effectively with Kaiser there. Thus we do not have to rely entirely on prepaid group practices for cost control. These other models of alternative delivery system, and even a traditional insurance carrier, can cut costs to compete if they must. Altogether, I believe it reasonable to estimate that a comprehensive system of fair economic competition of alternative delivery systems would eventually deliver the care people want for at least 25 percent less than the cost under today's system dominated by insured fee for service. And the care would be more satisfactory to consumers as well.

Although competition may work slowly and imperfectly, it is much more promising than the alternative—direct government controls, which are the subject of Chapter 6.

6
Why Price Controls and Similar Controls Don't Reduce Health Care Costs

REGULATION AS A SUBSTITUTE FOR APPROPRIATE ECONOMIC INCENTIVES[1]

The fundamental strategic choice for public policy on health care costs is competition or regulation. In Chapter 5 we saw how competition can change the basic structure and underlying incentives of our health care financing and delivery system. The subject of this chapter is regulation, by which I mean direct government controls over prices, capacity, and the use of services.

This is not a choice as to whether or not the government has a role to play in health care. Either way, the government must play an important part. As explained in Chapter 5, procompetitive regulation is needed to make the market work to achieve society's goals. Even the stock market, which economists consider to be a "perfect market," is supported by a great deal of procompetitive regulation, administered mainly by the Securities and Exchange Commission. Antitrust laws and laws prescribing fair-trade practices are generally accepted as a necessary support to our market economy. Procompetitive regulation is especially needed in the market for health care financing and delivery plans, in which we cannot have a completely free market, for reasons explained in Chapter 5.

Some forms of economic competition are undesirable, and society may have a good reason for ruling them out. For example, nobody recommends that we have a competition among unsafe airlines. We have extensive safety regulation of airlines administered by the Federal Aviation

93

Administration. "Deregulation of the airlines" meant abolition of the Civil Aeronautics Board's control over prices and routes flown, not abolition of the FAA. Similarly, I believe that abolition of physician licensure or hospital safety regulation would be a mistake. We don't need competition from unqualified doctors or unsafe hospitals. (However, the details of the restrictions on substitution of nonphysician personnel and the costs versus benefits of specific safety-code provisions deserve careful scrutiny.)

The choice between competition and regulation is a choice about the role of government. In the strategy of competition the government takes a much simpler and less intrusive role than in the regulatory approach. It seeks to set the basic framework of rules and incentives in such a way that the market (that is, the interaction of people making transactions in their own best interests) will produce the desired result. In the regulatory approach applied to health care, the government takes on a much more complex and demanding role, a role in which, in my view, it is bound to fail. In the regulatory approach government would leave today's cost-increasing incentives in place and then try to stop them from having their natural effect by direct detailed controls such as telling doctors how much they can charge for each service. In this approach direct controls are intended to substitute for rational economic incentives. In my view, the regulatory approach is like trying to make water run uphill, whereas in the competitive market approach the government is merely trying to channel the stream in its downhill course.

Procompetitive regulation is likely to be much simpler and more effective than direct controls on prices, capacity, and use of services, which act in opposition to the financial incentives. For in this case the basic incentives are pointing people in about the right direction. The regulators are attempting merely to modify the behavior of the regulated at the margin. Regulated entities would derive little financial benefit from changing or evading the rules. As a result, there are fewer, less ferociously battled attempts to do so. It isn't a life-and-death matter to beat the rules.

A good example of procompetitive regulation is the limitation on "insider trading" by officers of companies whose stock is traded on the stock exchanges. Officers of such companies are not allowed to profit from both buying and selling stock in their companies within a six-month interval. The purpose of the rule is to prevent people from taking unfair advantage of "insider information." If anyone profits from violation of this rule, the company is supposed to collect the profit from the violator. In case it does not, any shareholder is allowed to sue in the name of the company and, if successful, will be awarded part of the profits the violator made from the illegal trading. Enforcement of the rule is not a major problem for the government, in part because enforcement is done by private individuals and in part because there are plenty of legitimate ways that company officers can make profits without violating it.

Similarly, a rule requiring health plans to practice community rating would be relatively simple and easy to enforce. There would be some attempts to evade it, but evasion wouldn't do a health plan much good unless it were on such a large scale as to be obvious. And the economic pressures on health plans to evade the rule would not be large. There would be plenty of ways for a health plan to succeed without violating this rule.

On the other hand, under the regulatory approach, the regulators are attempting to make regulated entities behave in ways that are directly opposed to their financial interests, possibly even threatening their survival. Therefore, the incentive to attempt to bend, fight, or evade the regulations is much stronger. Medicare limits on hospital routine daily costs can mean millions of dollars in lost revenue. They cause delegations of hospital administrators and trustees to descend on their representatives in Congress. And they inspire the development of ingenious accounting strategies to shift costs to other categories. Limits on physician fees are met by numerous strategies by which physicians maintain their incomes. The efforts to change or to evade the regulations force regulators to deal with many individual cases. They subject regulators to continuing pressures to grant exceptions. This makes for even more complex regulations. Government is forced to involve itself in the details of more and more transactions. Rules that are simple in concept at the outset become extremely complex in application. And in the end, in health care the regulations generally fail to overcome the force of the cost-increasing incentives.[2] This chapter reviews the record of direct economic controls in the health services industry.

PRICE CONTROLS ON HOSPITALS: HOSPITAL-COST CONTAINMENT

On August 15, 1971, President Nixon announced Phase I of his Economic Stabilization Program, a ninety-day freeze on all wages and prices. The application to hospitals was ambiguous because much of hospital revenue is based on reimbursement of costs, not on prices charged, and such reimbursements did not fit neatly into the price-control model. Phase II regulations, published in December 1971, put a ceiling on hospital aggregate wage and salary increases of 5.5 percent per year, on aggregate nonwage and salary expense increases of 2.5 percent, and on aggregate expenses from "new technology" of 1.7 percent. Increases in aggregate revenue due to price increases were limited to 6 percent. Application of the rules was ambiguous because the appropriate unit of output on the basis of which to measure price or cost was not clear. Was it a day in the hospital? Or a stay in the hospital? Or each of the many individual services that hospitals perform? Ultimately, the regulators chose a compromise between cost per day and cost per admission. Many requests for exceptions ensued. Exceptions were granted routinely if adherence to the regulations would cause a hospital to suffer a net cash outflow.[3]

Phase III extended Phase II from January to June 1973. Final Phase IV regulations for health care, issued in January 1974, limited total charges and expenses per admission to an annual increase of no more than 7.5 percent and prescribed adjustments for changes in volume. The price controls ended on April 30, 1974, with expiration of the legislative authority on which they were based

What was the effect of thirty-two months of freezes and price controls? There was a slowdown in hospital spending. Paul Ginsburg, Ph.D., then a health services researcher at Duke University and now at the Congressional Budget Office, estimated that real (net of general inflation) expenditures per hospital admission increased 3.7 percent per year from the second quarter of 1971 to the second quarter of 1973, compared with an increase of 4.6 percent per year during a similar period from 1969 to 1971.[4] He estimated that growth in real expenditures per patient day slowed from 6.6 percent per year in the earlier period to 5.6 percent in the control period. The question is whether this was merely a continuation of a preexisting trend or whether the slowdown could be attributed to the price controls.

There have been two studies of the question. Each tried to estimate what the trend in hospital expenses would have been in the absence of controls and to compare that with what actually occurred. The results were ambiguous; they certainly did not demonstrate that the price controls were effective. Ginsburg found that "the Economic Stabilization Program was very effective in reducing rates of increase of hospital employees' wages, but not with regard to hospital costs."[5] (The whole control program was focused on moderating the rate of wage increase in all sectors.) The controls either had no effect or appeared to increase costs when measured on a per-patient-day basis. They appeared to reduce cost when measured on a per-admission basis. And the latter favorable effect disappeared if one assumed that the decrease in average length of hospital stay that took place during this period was not a result of the controls. (Since the incentives produced by the controls were to reward increasing length of stay, this is a reasonable assumption.)

The other study was done by Vanderbilt University economists Frank Sloan and Bruce Steinwald.[6] Using a longer time span and a broader data base than Ginsburg did, they attempted to measure the effect of the Economic Stabilization Program (and many other controls on hospitals) on total expense and labor expense per patient day and per admission. The results seemed to contradict each other. By most measures, the Economic Stabilization Program seemed to have a cost-increasing effect. The most favorable finding was that a year of these controls would reduce total expense per admission by two-thirds of one percent per year, compared with what they would be in the absence of controls, but even this was contradicted by other findings.

The question of what is the appropriate unit of output is of more than mere technical significance. If the authorities control hospital cost per day, they create an incentive for the hospital to increase length of stay and aggregate spending, because the later days in the hospital stay are typically less costly than the earlier days. If the authorities attempt to control hospital cost per admission (cost per case rather than per day), they create an incentive for a hospital—working through its medical staff—to admit more low cost cases that might otherwise have been cared for on an outpatient basis. Indeed, an economical organized system of care would be likely to have a high cost per day because it admits to the hospital only patients who really need to be there and keeps them in the hospital for only as long as necessary. Thus price-control programs can, and often do, have unintended side effects. Moreover, because the need for health care services is so much a matter of judgment, prices charged for individual services may bear little relation to total per capita cost of care. Yet this total is presumably what we are really seeking to control.

In April 1977 the Carter administration proposed its Hospital Cost Containment Act, which would have limited the annual increase in each hospital's inpatient revenue to a uniform percentage calculated by a formula based on overall inflation in the economy and the rate of increase in total hospital spending in the previous two years. The purpose was to slow the rate of growth in hospital spending down to the general rate of inflation in the economy. The bill included prescribed adjustments for significant volume changes and for numerous exceptions. The most important exception was a "wage pass-through," meaning that wage increases for nonsupervisory personnel above the percentage limit would not be counted in calculating a hospital's spending increase. This illustrates the kind of political concession needed to pass such legislation. Hospital workers are now paid as much as people with equal education and experience doing similar jobs elsewhere. Since wages account for a large part of hospital costs, this "pass-through" would have weakened the controls a great deal. A modified version of this bill was passed in the Senate, but failed in the House of Representatives.

The administration tried again in March 1979. Although similar in general concept to the earlier proposal, the second bill contained several differences from the first one. First, the mandatory controls would become effective only if a "national voluntary limit" on hospital inpatient revenue increases of 9.7 percent was exceeded and then only in the states that exceeded the limit. Second, the mandatory limit would be equal to the sum of the increase in an index of the prices of goods and services hospitals buy, plus a 1.8 percent allowance for population growth and new services. Third, there would be an "efficiency/inefficiency allowance." Hospitals would be grouped by size and location into "peer groups." Hospitals with "routine costs per day" (board and routine nursing costs) less than 90 percent of the median for their group would be allowed an additional 1 percent annual increase. Hospitals between 90 and 100 percent would be allowed an additional 0.5 percent growth. Hospitals with routine costs over 115 percent of the group median would be penalized a percentage point. Again, many exceptions would be allowed, including the "wage pass-through." During the summer of 1979, the Carter administration accepted one after another provision that would weaken the controls, such as a "sunset" clause, until the bill had become little more than a symbolic act. The bill was voted down by the House of Representatives in November 1979.

In defending its 1979 proposal, the Carter administration appealed to the experience of nine states with mandatory hospital-cost controls. These states averaged a 12.1 percent increase in total hospital costs in 1977, compared with 16.8 percent for states without such controls. Have state controls been successful? If so, would a similar national program be successful?

The evidence on the first question is equivocal. The Sloan and Steinwald study is the only one that has attempted to control statistically for the many relevant variables. And its data ended with 1975. The findings were mixed—some favorable and some unfavorable—to the efficacy of state controls on hospital spending. The most favorable finding would imply that if payment for all patients were subject to controls, in the long run hospital costs would be 4.8 percent lower than without controls.

Paul Ginsburg and Lawrence Wilson at the Congressional Budget Office did a much simpler analysis of cost growth from 1976 to 1978, controlling statistically for fewer variables.[7] They found that mandatory state hospital-spending controls reduced the annual growth rate of expenditures by three percentage points. Whether or not all of this difference can be attributed to controls is not clear. Spending in the more costly states grew more slowly than spending in the less costly states. And most of the states with mandatory state controls were among the most costly. This could explain a substantial part of the difference.

The state in which hospital-rate controls appear to have had the most effect is New York. Its hospital expenditures per capita were 148 percent of the national average in 1969, when the state control program began, and 135 percent in 1977. In both years it was the second most costly state. On the other hand, controls had little or no apparent effect in some other states. For example, per capita spending in New Jersey was 88 percent of the national average when its control program began in 1971 and 92 percent in 1977. Maryland's per capita hospital spending was 93 percent of the national average in 1973 and 91 percent in 1977, not a very large improvement.

It seems doubtful that a national program of mandatory controls would be as effective as the controls were in these few states. New York was in quite special circumstances. The state was in a financial crisis to which Medicaid was a major contributor. The political will to act was there. Congressional reception to the Carter proposals does not suggest that there is a similar will to act at the national level. There is an important element of self-selection. Controls are less likely to work well in states where they are imposed involuntarily than in states that adopt them on their own. And most of the states with apparently effective controls are among the most costly, where there is more fat easier to cut.

The main thing wrong with the proposed Hospital Cost Containment Act was that it contained nothing to correct the perverse incentives in our dominant financing system. It contained nothing to help basic reform of the financing and delivery system. It was a pure spending restraint that reflected no concern for health care quality, efficiency, or equity. There is no good reason to suppose that its effects would be focused on reduction in waste as opposed to reduction in spending in general. On the contrary, this kind of control reinforces the cost-increasing incentives. In the face of such a control system, a hospital that thought that it could get by one year with less than the allowed increase in revenues would be foolish to take less. To do so would diminish its "entitlement" to future increases. (Hospitals that think that they need more than the allowed increase would apply for exceptions.)

The original Carter administration proposal clearly would have rewarded the fat and punished the lean. Imagine two hospitals doing exactly the same job, one for $1 million a year, the other for $2 million. An equal percentage increase allows the latter an increase of twice the dollar amount. In recognition of this problem, the 1979 proposal included the "efficiency/inefficiency bonus/penalty" described above, but it too had several things wrong with it. To begin with, routine costs per day are a very poor proxy for "efficiency." Indeed, most of the factors responsible for the unjustified increase in costs, such as overuse of and overinvestment in costly specialized facilities, are not counted in routine cost per day.

Furthermore, the administration's proposal admitted that "data do not yet exist for classifying hospitals by type of patients cared for," a necessary ingredient for a satisfactory comparison of hospital costs. The lack of a suitable classification is not the result of a lack of trying to find one. This problem will not be solved soon. Developing a reliable method for classifying the severity of illness of a hospital's patients is one of the toughest unsolved problems in health services research. A low hospital cost per day does not necessarily mean efficiency; it may instead reflect the fact that too many hospitalized patients are not really sick.

This system is sure to lead to endless complex arguments as to which hospitals are suitable peers. When Medicare introduced a similar concept, many people flew to Washington to explain why they should be included in a different market area, why they should be given credit for the severity of the cases they treated, and so forth. There is nothing as unique as a hospital!

The formula included in the administration proposal would not have worked very quickly to narrow the disparities between the "efficient" and the "inefficient." Consider two "peer" hospitals, one with a routine cost of $90 per day and the other with a routine cost of $115, compared with a peer-group mean of $100. Assume, as the administration did, that the basic controlled rate of growth would have been 9.7 percent. Then, if the low-cost hospital took its allowed 9.7 percent, plus its 0.5 percent efficiency bonus while the high-cost hospital increased at its allowed 9.7 percent, at the end of five years the costs would be $146.27 and $182.70, respectively. The former would have gone from 78 percent of the latter to 80 percent, hardly an overwhelming "bonus."

Thus the 1979 Carter proposal would still have rewarded the fat and punished the lean. Such an effect is inherent in this type of control system. Moreover, as noted earlier, controlling cost per admission introduces more perverse incentives. Hospitals that wanted to beat the system could increase total spending faster while holding down cost per admission by encouraging their medical staffs to admit more low-cost, less seriously ill cases or "cycling" patients in and out of the hospital. Some hospitals would seek to avoid the impact of the revenue limit by "unbundling" services. That is, they might have some services performed on an outpatient basis to people who previously would have been treated on an inpatient basis, to get these services out from under the inpatient revenue limit, and then encourage the admission of other patients. Or, they might switch the billing, if not the provision, of services from the hospital to the doctor. Some physicians might redirect the flow of patients from hospitals under mandatory controls to other hospitals still below their revenue limits. The possibilities are endless. Would-be regulators reply that they will develop countermeasures to detect and punish such behavior. Inevitably, this will elicit countercountermeasures, and so on, until the system bogs down in complexity.

When viewed realistically in our present political context, "hospital-cost containment" seems unlikely to be effective. As well as the above problems with incentives, there is the problem that hospitals would almost inevitably be exempted from the controls once the controls threatened to cause bankruptcy. Barring an unusual financial crisis, as in New York, few regulators will be willing to bear the onus of driving hospitals into bankruptcy. Thus once a hospital's expenses rise to equal the allowed revenues, the price controls become, in effect, a system of cost reimbursement, with all of the cost increases being allowed and "passed through." By contrast, one of the great virtues of the private competitive market is its impersonal character. If price controls threaten to drive a hospital into bankruptcy, the hospital can appeal and bring political pressure to bear on the regulators. If, instead, a system of economic competition were created and allowed to function, the inefficient hospital facing bankruptcy would have no one to pressure. It would have to cut costs or risk being driven out of business.

All this is not to say that given the requisite laws and political will, a regulatory system could not possibly limit the rate of growth in hospital costs. A system that is sufficiently tough and comprehensive could do the job. In effect, the government would be controlling the budget of each hospital. Rather, it is to say that given our values and our political system as it actually operates, such an effective cost-containment program seems unlikely. But even if such a control program were effective in controlling the aggregate growth of hospital expenditures, it would have done nothing to improve the efficiency of hospitals, the quality of their services, or the equity with which those services are distributed. The likely outcome would be a uniform percentage growth in the spending of each hospital. Each hospital, whether well managed or poorly managed, whether serving the most urgent needs or not, would be assured an annual budget increase. The hospital industry would be frozen into its present patterns.

The general history of economic regulation in our country does not support the presumption that regulation reduces costs to consumers. Indeed, the present moves to deregulate transportation are based on powerful evidence that regulation has raised costs.

How would the officials charged with controlling hospital budgets avoid "capture by the regulated"—a fate all too common in other regulated industries? Why should these regulators hold down the costs and take the political heat from outraged local interest groups? There would be no reward for them in doing so. If they do an effective job, the hospitals will bring pressure to bear on the legislators who have oversight over the regulators, and the legislators will put the heat on the regulators to force them to be more compliant. If the regulators deviate too far from the wishes of the hospitals, the hospitals may lead a campaign to get the regulatory system abolished, as they did, successfully, in Colorado.

Finally, one of the main arguments used in support of hospital-cost containment was that it could be effective quickly. The alternative of fundamental delivery-system reform was dismissed on the grounds that "it would take too long, and we can't wait." But the history of such controls does not support the view that they work quickly. In 1977 Harold A. Cohen, Executive Director of the Maryland Health Services Cost Review Commission, created by a law enacted in 1971 and one of the oldest and best publicized of the state hospital cost-control agencies, wrote: "It is much too early to say whether public utility-type regulation of hospitals can work. . . . It is clear that many problems have surfaced. . . . Yet the current system cannot be fine tuned. It must be completely overhauled if costs are to be contained."[8]

HEALTH PLANNING AND CERTIFICATE OF NEED

Starting with New York in 1965, states have been enacting certificate-of-need (CON) laws, under which a regulatory authority must issue a permit based on assessment of needs in the area before an increase in hospital capacity can occur. By mid-1974, twenty-four states had enacted some form of CON statute. That year, Congress passed the National Health Planning and Resources Development Act. The main effect of the act has been to create a national regulatory structure to be based on 206 "health systems agencies," local regulatory bodies, and 50 state health-planning and development agencies. Among other things, health systems agencies are supposed to provide effective "health planning" for their areas in order to increase the accessibility and quality of health services, restrain cost increases, and prevent unnecessary duplication of health resources. The act required each state to enact a CON law by 1980 or lose certain federal funds. The federal budget for 1980 included $209 million to support health planning, but the actual cost of this activity is much larger because this appropriation does not pay for the large costs incurred by hospitals in complying with the law.

Several broadly based studies comparing states with and without certificate-of-need programs have concluded that CON has failed to ameliorate the problem of hospital overinvestment. For example, the Washington-based consulting firm Lewin and Associates found that thirty of forty-one states and areas that had such controls in 1974 and for which data could be obtained "approved hospital beds in excess of 105 per cent of their published need projection for five years hence. Fourteen of these began the period overbedded and approved additional beds; five others became overbedded during the period studied as a result of the projects they approved."[9]

David Salkever and Thomas Bice, Professors of Health Services at Johns Hopkins and the University of Washington, respectively, did a statistical analysis of the impact of CON controls on hospital investment between 1966 and 1972.[10] Their results indicate that CON controls did not reduce the total dollar amount of investment, but they did alter its composition by reducing growth in beds and increasing other types of investments. Social Security Administration economist Fred Hellinger did a similar study and found that CON legislation "has not significantly lowered hospital investment and that hospitals anticipated the effect of CON legislation by increasing investment in the period preceding the enactment of the legislation."[11] Sloan and Steinwald found that the anticipation of CON had a significant cost-increasing impact.[12] The certificate-of-need programs themselves had either essentially no impact on hospital costs or a cost-increasing effect. No statistically controlled studies have reached the opposite conclusion.

Why has CON proved to be so ineffective? There are several reasons. Depending on the circumstances, there may be little or no incentive for ordinary citizens serving on a health systems agency board to turn down a proposed project. Why should they vote to deny approval when it would mean jobs and improved services in the local area, paid for in large part by state and federal taxpayers in general (through Medicaid and Medicare) and by employers and insurance carriers whose tax-subsidized premiums reflect costs over a wider area? Hospitals tend to have their own constituencies. One is the pride of the Catholic community, another of the Lutherans, and so forth. Prominent citizens serve on their boards. Like other people, regulators like to avoid conflicts and to produce successes. The opening ceremony for a beautiful new hospital wing is a happy occasion for civic leaders. The rewards for denying approval are far less tangible, if they exist at all.

Nobody knows how to do "health planning." There is a general lack of good data and an almost complete lack of criteria for evaluating the need for health facilities. Consider as basic a concept as the appropriate number of hospital beds for a community. Regulators cannot simply look at how many beds are used or unused, because there is no reason to believe that the way things are is the way they should be. To produce a standard, regulators would have to determine what bed use would be if all patients were given optimal medical care. Because this is subject to such wide variations in opinion among physicians, reaching a consensus on this issue, particularly one that is very different from the status quo, would be all but impossible. This was illustrated by the Committee on Controlling the Supply of Short-Term General Hospital Beds of the Institute of Medicine of the National Academy of Sciences, a balanced group of leading health care experts. After five years of study, the committee was unable to reach agreement on a standard for community bed needs. Under pressure applied through the chairman, the committee was finally able to agree that the existing supply of 4.4 beds per 1000 people ought to be reduced by at least 10 percent within the next five years, with further significant reductions thereafter.[13] The committee could not agree on a standard that would have any measurable impact on hospitalization. The Department of Health, Education, and Welfare subsequently converted this number into a planning guideline of 4.0 beds per 1000 people. In view of the fact that the large prepaid group practices owning hospitals operate at about 1.5 beds per 1000 (which would be closer to 2.0 if they cared for a representative population mix), the inability of the committee to set a standard below 4.0 left much room for disagreement and doubt about what the number should be.

Even measuring the existing number of beds per 1000 population is not without its problems. Should the ratio refer to licensed beds (which may be mere pieces of paper without tangible counterparts), to existing beds (which may not be in usable condition or staffed), or to staffed and available beds? If the latter, precisely how is "availability" defined and ascertained? If such difficulties surround such a comparatively simple notion as the ratio of short-term hospital beds to population, consider how much more difficult it would be to regulate effectively the hundreds of different technologies that are used in a modern hospital every day.

The best the regulatory authorities might hope to do is to eliminate obvious excess capacity by denying new construction permits and letting population catch up with existing capacity. It seems unlikely that they would deny capacity needed to care for people whose doctors say they need it. The key opportunities for cutting cost by curtailing "flat-of-the-curve" use of services are not addressed by certificate-of-need regulation.

But the research results seem to suggest something worse than ineffectiveness. Could CON raise costs? Aside from the obvious costs of paperwork and delay, researchers have noted several perverse side effects. For one, the anticipation of CON has triggered building and buying booms, in the expectation that projects on order before the law became effective would be "grandfathered." In the face of uncertainty about future needs and permission to meet them, institutions have an incentive to overstate needs and to "stockpile" capacity. Institutions that have excess capacity that they would otherwise retire from service are reluctant to do so, for fear that they will then lose their licenses and be unable to put the capacity back in operation when they need it. CON has in some cases created a paper franchise value for hospital bed licenses. In one example the owners of a hospital that would have cost some $9 million to replace demanded a price in excess of $30 million from a growing HMO that needed more beds, simply because it appeared that the HMO would be unable to get CON approval to build its own hospital in an overbedded area. (Fortunately, the law has been changed to exempt hospitals that serve mostly HMO members.)

Furthermore, the certificate-of-need process can stop only new investments. The health systems agencies do not have, and are not likely to obtain, the authority to shut down existing underused or inefficient facilities. The effect is to protect existing providers from competition from new cost-reducing innovators and to force the efficient to subsidize the inefficient. The trouble, of course, is that this further diminishes any incentive to improve efficiency.

How all this works in an actual case is illustrated by the staff analysis of the West Bay Health Systems Agency, San Francisco, in support of its recommendation to deny approval to Kaiser-Permanente to establish its own open-heart surgery unit at one of its hospitals.[14] Kaiser had been buying open-heart surgery services from outside hospitals, mainly Stanford University Medical Center. In April 1978 Kaiser applied for a CON to open its own unit. The application projected that the unit would perform 330 operations in its first year, enough to make it proficient and economical. (Recall the discussion in Chapter 3.) Kaiser projected that its savings would be $2 million in the first full year of operation, growing to $3.7 million per year four years later.

The health systems agency recommended that the Kaiser application be denied because the existing heart surgery facilities would not cut back their spending if Kaiser stopped referring patients to them. Therefore, the overall effect of Kaiser's establishing its own unit would be to increase total cost. The agency observed:

> There is little chance that in the short run, the current capacity of the open-heart surgery facilities will be reduced and potentially inappropriate or more costly less efficient facilities phased out. The reimbursement mecha-

nism enables fee-for-service hospitals to pass on cost increases to third-party payors and thus avoid possible operating deficits due to inefficiencies. Furthermore, the HSA does not have authority to close low volume high cost facilities although it can recommend to the State of California to do so. [The report included no such recommendation.] . . . As is true in many regulatory issues, what appears good for an individual provider is not necessarily good for the community. . . . Kaiser in a sense is being penalized for desiring to expand in a situation where both high cost providers and excess capacity exist.[15]

The problem is not with the agency's personnel, who understood the situation and doubtless would have preferred to see some of the low-volume high-cost facilities closed. Rather, the problem is in the nature of this type of regulation.

In other words, in this kind of regulatory system the efficient innovator must yield to the inefficient established providers. It should not be surprising that such a system adds to cost. In a fair competitive market system with prudent buyers conscious of both cost and quality, it is the inefficient low-volume providers who would be driven out of business.

CONTROLS ON PHYSICIANS' FEES

Close behind price controls on hospitals, on the regulatory agenda, are controls on physicians' fees. The Carter administration's National Health Plan, proposed in the spring of 1979, included such controls. Initially, physicians serving Medicare and Medicaid patients would be required to accept as full payment fees based on average Medicare physician-payment levels. Subsequent fee schedules would be negotiated between the government and physician representatives. Private health insurance plans would be "encouraged" to use these official fees also.

We have had limited experience with government controls on physician fees. Medicaid programs have set their own limits, with the effect that many physicians refuse to participate in Medicaid. Medicare has "fee screens," or limits on what it considers to be "usual, customary, and reasonable (UCR)." Because these limits are often substantially less than what physicians actually charge, Medicare beneficiaries often find that 80 percent of what Medicare considers "UCR" is a much lower percentage of their actual doctor bill. Thus the effect of a partial control system can be either to deny services to beneficiaries or to shift costs onto them, rather than to control costs.

Our only experience with comprehensive controls on physicians' fees occurred during the Nixon administration's Economic Stabilization Program. In August 1971 fees were frozen for ninety days, but subsequently were allowed to rise at prescribed rates. For example, in Phase IV a physician could not raise the aggregate of all of his or her fees by more than 4 percent per year and could not raise any individual fee by more than 10 percent. What were the consequences? Any analysis of this question is limited by the fact that data on physicians' incomes and the prices they charge are quite unreliable. For example, the consumer price index tends to reflect what physicians announce as their "customary fees" and not what they actually get, net of discounts and bad debts. Nevertheless, such data as exist suggest the following conclusions.

The Economic Stabilization Program did slow the growth in physicians' fees. Before the controls, they were growing faster than the overall consumer price index (CPI). During 1972 and 1973, they grew at a rate slower than consumer prices in general. In 1971 they grew 6.9 percent, compared with 4.3 percent for the CPI. In 1972 and 1973 they grew 3.1 and 3.3 percent, compared with 3.3 and 6.2 percent in the CPI. Thus they were reduced in real terms.

The price controls also stopped the growth in real per capita spending on physicians' services. In fact, in constant 1967 dollars (that is, deflated by the CPI), 1974 per capita spending on physicians' services was $59.90, compared with $59.40 in 1971 and $61.98 in 1972.[16] However, the volume of physicians' services increased by almost enough to offset the decline in the real value of physicians' fees. Economist Zachary Dyckman described it this way in a report for the Council on Wage and Price Stability:

> It is interesting to note that the greatest two-year change in physicians' services occurred during the two-year period when price controls were in effect, FY 1973 and FY 1974. [FY refers to the fiscal years of the federal government, then running from June to June.] While fees, as measured by the CPI, rose 2.4 and 4.0 percent, respectively, during FY 1973 and FY 1974, physician utilization increased 6.3 and 5.5 percent respectively. It is possible that physicians may have increased their services to sustain a pattern of increasing income levels. Or, perhaps, they redefined services so that prices could be implicitly rather than explicitly increased. . . . However, the substantial increase in measured utilization during only those years when price controls were in effect and the subsequent resumption of more normal patterns of utilization increases suggest that physicians may have increased billings to compensate for their inability to raise fees above that level allowed under the controls program. This view is supported by recent research.[17]

In other words, because physicians can, and apparently did, control the volume of services provided for a given medical condition, they can easily evade the controls if the purpose of the controls is to limit spending on their services.

Finally, the median net income of physicians increased during this period by about the same percentage as the CPI. What can these experiences tell us about the likely success of controls on physicians' fees as a contributor to overall cost control? For one thing, such controls are addressed to a comparatively small part of the total problem of health care costs. As noted earlier, physicians' gross incomes account for about 18 percent of the grand total. In view of the key role of physicians in determining the grand total, it would make more sense to enlist their support for economical use of health care resources in general rather than to attempt to reduce their incomes.

Moreover, prices are ratios, with dollars in the numerator and units of service in the denominator. Proposed controls on the prices physicians charge are based on the naive and false assumption that there is a stable and meaningful denominator. As we have seen, the "doctor visit" is not a precise or standard unit of service. Rather, it is almost infinitely compressible. A doctor whose income is threatened by price controls can cut the average length of his or her visits from fifteen minutes to five. Part of the problem is that in some circumstances, a half-minute visit might be quite appropriate from a medical point of view. Whether or not it is will be a matter of judgment, a judgment that a regulatory authority is very poorly placed to second-guess. Moreover, the need for doctor visits is impossible to evaluate objectively except in extreme cases. So the doctor can advise chronically ill patients to come back next week instead of next month. Doctors can also "unbundle," with separate fees for separate services performed on the same visit. An injection or the drawing of a blood sample that used to be included in the "routine office visit" fee can be billed separately. Doctors can upgrade the content of visits, turning what would have been a "routine visit" into a complicated procedure.

Canada has a national health insurance system in which physicians' fees are set by negotiation between physicians and provincial governments. In some years the governments have managed to hold down the increases in fees to rates below the rate of increase in the cost of living. From 1970 to 1975, the Canadian consumer price index increased 42 percent while physicians' fees increased 17 percent. Physicians' net incomes increased 32 percent, indicating that physicians, using all of the methods described above, were able to protect themselves at least in substantial part, if not completely.

In reviewing this experience, Robert Evans, a Canadian economist, observed:

> Control in the existing structure includes negotiation of list fees. . . . The evidence now seems fairly clear that this will not work because billings can be expanded almost indefinitely on a given schedule. Moreover, procedural multiplication can be harmful to the patient's health and can generate substantial external costs in the hospital sector and elsewhere. The "provider profiles" mentioned above [a statistical screening device] merely identify very unusual practitioners. They give no leverage to government over changes in medical practice standards over time. A variety of gimmicks have been suggested or tried. For example, absolute limits on physician earnings (Newfoundland) merely lead to more physician leisure. Prorationing of bills against a fixed pool of reimbursement has been suggested as a short run measure, but in the long run it seems to accentuate the pressures on physicians to multiply procedures by penalizing the "non-multipliers" for the excesses of their colleagues.[18]

Government controls on physicians' fees can have other perverse effects. One effect of a freeze is to reward those doctors who raised their fees early and who charge high prices and to penalize those who did the opposite. A particular danger in the type of controls used by the Nixon administration is that they can damage or destroy the ability of HMOs to compete for physicians. HMO physicians are much more vulnerable to controls than are fee-for-service physicians because they offer comprehensive care for an all-inclusive payment. Thus HMO physicians cannot make up the loss from price controls by increased volume, "unbundling," or similar tactics.

Perhaps the worst effect of the kind of negotiated-fee schedule proposed by both the Carter administration and Senator Kennedy (see Appendix) is that it would unite the doctors in opposition to the government. Considering the urgent nature of the need for some medical care, that is a negotiation in which the doctors are likely to have considerable power. It seems highly likely that they would be able to "lock in" fees close, in real terms, to those prevailing today. A more sensible goal for public policy would be to encourage the organization of doctors into competing economic units. A negotiated-fee schedule would be a major step away from such competition.

UTILIZATION REVIEW AND PROFESSIONAL STANDARDS REVIEW ORGANIZATIONS

Since the mid-1960s, hospitals participating in Medicare and Medicaid have been required to have a utilization review plan, with committees and procedures for reviewing the appropriateness of the use of hospital services by beneficiaries of these programs. The purpose is to curtail unnecessary hospital use. In 1972 the Senate Finance Committee expressed alarm over the very large cost overruns in Medicare and Medicaid. Among the causes "the committee has found that present utilization review requirements and activities are not adequate. A significant proportion of the health services provided under Medicare and Medicaid are probably not medically necessary."[19] So the committee included in its 165 pages of amendments to the Social Security Act a section directing the Secretary of Health, Education, and Welfare to create a national system of Professional Standards Review Organizations (PSROs).

A PSRO was to be an independent, nonprofit association of physicians, broadly representative of the practicing physicians in each local area, with the competence to provide medical review services:

A PSRO would have the responsibility of determining—for purposes of eligibility for Medicare and Medicaid reimbursement—whether care and services provided were: first, medically necessary, and second, provided in accordance with professional standards. Additionally, the PSRO, where medically appropriate, would encourage the attending physician to utilize less costly alternative sites and modes of treatment.[20]

The PSRO would be expected to use automated screening of claims, registered nurses, and other review personnel to assist physicians in identifying questionable cases and would be required to delegate responsibility to hospital review committees when such committees could demonstrate effective capacity to do the reviewing.

The secretary divided the nation into 203 "PSRO areas." By April 1977, ninety-six areas had active PSROs performing "concurrent review" of hospital use. The program was supported by DHEW at a cost of about $150 million per year. Although the law also referred to concerns over quality, it is very clear from the law and committee reports that the main purpose of the PSROs was cost control. However, the establishment and effectiveness of PSROs was clearly dependent on the acceptance and support of the medical profession. And in developing and selling the program, DHEW shifted the emphasis from cost control to quality assurance in order to make it more palatable to doctors.[21]

Have the PSROs been effective in controlling cost? The possibility of a scientifically sound evaluation has been impaired by the lack of an experimental approach to the program, by poor data, and by the already existing downward trends in hospital use in some areas before PSROs were established. There have been many evaluations of individual PSROs or similar review organizations with other names. For example, a RAND Corporation team did a detailed statistical evaluation of four years of experience of the New Mexico Experimental Medical Care Review Organization and found that "the medical review system produced no net savings, nor did it have a demonstrable effect on hospital use."[22] They also reviewed the literature on PSRO effectiveness and reported: "Most studies attempted to evaluate changes produced by complicated (utilization review) strategies in different areas of the country. In a few cases the results supported (utilization review) effectiveness; in most cases they did not. . . . Most programs apparently produced little or no net dollar savings."[23]

The most firmly based analyses were done by the Health Care Financing Administration (HCFA)—the branch of DHEW that administers Medicare and Medicaid—in 1978 and by Paul Ginsburg and Daniel Koretz of the Congressional Budget Office in 1979.[24] Both compared 1977 hospital use per person in the ninety-six areas in which PSROs had become active by April 1977 with use in ninety-three areas without active PSROs. (The comparisons made allowance for use in the pre-PSRO year 1974 and for numerous other factors thought to affect hospital use.) HCFA concluded that PSROs reduced hospital use some 1.5 percent and that the savings they generated exceeded their costs by about 10 percent. Using somewhat different methods, Ginsburg and Koretz estimated that PSROs reduced hospital use 2 percent, but that the savings realized were 30 percent less than the cost of the PSRO program. Thus even the more optimistic HCFA estimate implied that the net savings to the Medicare program attributable to PSROs were about one-tenth of 1 percent of the costs of Medicare! Despite the large problems in making such estimates with any precision, what emerges clearly from all of the studies is the lack of evidence that PSROs have made any substantial contribution to cost control.

Why has the PSRO program been such a failure? The main reason is that like the other regulatory systems, it leaves the cost-increasing incentives of insured fee for service intact. It may even reinforce them. A physician is likely to feel much more vulnerable to charges of providing too little than too much care. The consequences of too little care are medically palpable; those of too much are medically quite abstract, though economically real. Why should a doctor who believes that the length of stay for uncomplicated heart attack patients could be cut safely from fourteen to seven days stand up to colleagues who do not want to make the change?

If a PSRO were effective, it would reduce the revenues of local providers, and the savings would revert to the government. There is no budget or "tradeoff" for the local providers: A dollar saved is a dollar lost. PSROs are entirely in the hands of local doctors, who have direct financial and professional interest in maintaining a high and costly standard of care.

The entire concept of PSROs rests on some of the naive notions criticized in Chapter 1, especially the idea that "for each medical condition, there is a 'best' treatment." Such standards, for the most part, do not and are not likely to exist. Medicine remains largely an art; it is not a branch of engineering. As a result, in practice, utilization review norms have become averages of actual practice rather than the results of systematic benefit-cost analysis. These statistical criteria can be used to identify those doctors who keep their patients in the hospital far more than average and to put pressure on them to depart less from the average. But this is unlikely to have much effect on physician behavior in general. Although reducing the use of resources by the most prodigal, it is also likely to increase the use of resources by the most frugal. This kind of system puts pressure on physicians to conform more closely to the norm. It doesn't contain any pressure to make the norm more economical.

The pattern that emerges from a review of these and other attempts at economic regulation of health care is an almost unbroken record of failure.

REGULATION VERSUS COMPETITION

The examples of competition described in Chapter 5 and the examples of regulation described in this chapter support some generalizations about the consequences of these two approaches to cost control when applied to health care.

Regulation often raises costs to consumers. Regulators become responsible for the economic survival of the regulated. If they let a regulated entity fail, they will be blamed for denying society a needed service and for causing a loss of jobs. So they cannot force the regulated to sustain losses or even to live with less than some target rate of return on investment. So cost increases have to be "passed through" to consumers, and price controls become cost reimbursement, with all of its cost-increasing incentives.

Regulators are often "captured" by the regulated. They must get their information about the regulated industry from the regulated. The regulated firms hire high-priced lawyers and lobbyists who exert a constant pressure in their favor. The consumer interest in lower prices or better service is too diffused to allow for an effectively organized counterpressure. The formal procedures of regulation also make it very costly and time-consuming. This is especially true if there are many entities to be regulated, with many special circumstances to be considered, as is the case with physicians and hospitals. All this helps explain why, for example, for many years, intrastate air travel, beyond the reach of the Civil Aeronautics Board, cost about half as much as interstate flights of the same length. Similarly, Interstate Commerce Commission regulation of trucking has added billions of dollars to the costs to customers.[25]

Competition, on the other hand, sets up an inexorable force for cost reduction. If company B can make a product of equal quality to company A's, but for less cost, it can sell it for a lower price and take the business away from company A. If company A cannot match the cost reduction, it will lose profits in the short run and risk being driven out of business in the long run. Survival demands that it cut costs. It has no regulators to appeal to for protection.

Regulation often retards beneficial innovation. Roger Noll, Professor of Economics at the California Institute of Technology, put it this way:

> Thwarting a promising innovation frequently occurs when a technological change threatens to shift substantial business from one regulated firm to another or to cause the profits of a regulated industry to decline. The Federal Communications Commission provides several examples of this behavior: the long standing prohibition (recently reversed) of foreign attachments—i.e., devices made by someone other than the American Telephone and Telegraph Company (AT&T)—to the switched telephone network; the decade-long delay in authorizing a domestic communications satellite; and the restrictions on the development of pay television and cable television. In all cases the new technology promises to offer new services that consumers have demonstrated a willingness to pay for, and old services at a substantial reduction in cost. . . . [but] the resources of the potential entrants for dealing with regulators, the Congress, and the courts are far fewer than those of the entrenched firms. . . .[26]

Noll's gloomy predictions about this impact of regulation in health care have been borne out by experience.

Competition rewards innovation and often channels it in socially desirable directions. Fortunes are made on new products and services, so innovations that lead to better services or reduced costs are encouraged. Firms that do not match their competitors' innovations often do not survive.

Market economies are the most effective in improving productivity and raising living standards. There are good reasons for this. People accept efficiency-improving changes such as closing unneeded plants or hospitals produced by impersonal market forces in the private sector. The people directly affected may not like them, but there is not much they can do about them. In the long run the whole economy benefits. But when such changes are imposed by government, those who would be harmed resist them, usually successfully, through legal and political action. Consider the extreme difficulty of closing unneeded post offices, defense installations, and Public Health Service hospitals. People will resist closing an underused post office and then turn around and complain about the cost and inefficiency of the postal system. It would be virtually impossible to close many unneeded hospitals by regulatory action—yet such closings are an important source of potential savings.

In market systems producers and consumers adapt continuously and gradually to changing conditions, even in anticipation of future events. The expectation of higher gasoline prices in the future motivates people to buy cars with good mileage now. In regulatory systems the rules themselves create vested interests which make the rules very difficult to change. These factors make for great rigidity in regulated industries, in contrast to flexible adaptation in markets.

Government often responds to well-focused producer interests; competitive markets respond systematically, if imperfectly, to consumer interests. Voters base their choices on issues of decisive personal importance, on their pocketbooks if they see their livelihoods at stake. People specialize in production and diversify in consumption. To a dairy farmer, a rise in coffee prices is a minor irritant, but an increase in the price of milk (supported by government) is a "make-or-break" issue. People are therefore much more likely to pressure their representatives about the issues that affect their livelihoods than on their interests as consumers, and their companies and unions provide natural organizations for doing so. In competitive markets companies get their revenues from satisfied customers who have alternative choices. So in product and pricing decisions, business must seek to serve the desires of consumers. Thus the choice between a regulated and a competitive market system of health care services is a choice between service that responds mainly to the interests of providers or to those of consumers.

Regulation depends on coercion, on forcing people to behave in ways they consider opposed to their own best interests. The decentralized competitive market, on the other hand, leaves maximum freedom to individual providers and consumers consistent with achievement of society's purposes. As Charles Schultze put it:

> Relationships in the market are a form of unanimous-consent arrangement. When dealing with each other in a buy-sell transaction, individuals can act voluntarily on the basis of mutual advantage. . . . Market-like arrangements not only minimize the need for coercion as a means of organizing society; they also reduce the need for compassion, patriotism, brotherly love, and cultural solidarity as motivating forces behind social improvement.[27]

The development of these desirable virtues is more likely to be encouraged if we do not place too heavy a burden on people who practice them. Moreover, the market encourages the pluralism and diversity that is valued by the American people. The regulatory approach works on the basis of uniform numerical standards.

Coercion and uniform standards are wasteful. They make economizing more costly and painful than it needs to be. The market approach allows people to make necessary adaptations in ways that are least costly or painful to themselves. For example, the President wanted us to save energy, so he issued an order that thermostats for air conditioning must be raised to 78°. The result was angry people and pleas for consideration of special circumstances. Groceries and restaurants need lower temperatures to preserve the food. Retailers of clothing need lower temperatures so that perspiring customers will not spoil the clothes they try on. Computers cannot operate at these temperatures, and so on. If, instead, the President were to use the market approach, he would find energy prices rising to equal the real cost of replacing that energy. All energy users would find it in their interest to economize. (The poor could be protected by appropriate subsidies based on income.) And each person could adapt in ways that suited his or her own circumstances best. Some would raise their thermostats to 78°. Some would turn off the air conditioning altogether. Others would keep the thermostats at 70°, but install insulation or heat-reflecting blinds on the windows or shorten the hours of operation. There are hundreds of ways to save energy, all of which would be tried if we let the market work. And by allowing the market to work, we would allow each person to adapt to the rising cost of energy in the way that discomforts him or her the least.

Some social arrangements persist because they make some people better off at the expense of other people. The regulation of health care promises to make practically everyone worse off than they would be in an economically rational market system. That such regulation has achieved so much acceptance must be explained, in part, by the fact that people have not understood how such a market system can be brought into existence. That is the subject of Chapter 7.

7

Consumer Choice
Health Plan

BACKGROUND

Consumer Choice Health Plan is my proposal for universal health insurance based on rational economic incentives and fair competition. Although it has drawn on many ideas, its main conceptual origins were in the early experience of the prepaid group practice plans that were seeking to be offered to members of employee groups after World War II. These plans were based on "closed panels," or a limited choice of doctor. Unless the plans could be virtually the unanimous choice of an employee group, the only way that they could hope to be offered was as an alternative to the traditional "free choice of doctor" insurance plan. Otherwise, to offer them, an employer would have had to take the unpopular step of limiting the employees' choice of doctor. At the time, "dual choice" was a radical idea in the world of health insurance.

By the late 1950s, when health insurance for federal employees was being considered, the prepaid group practices and the principle of dual choice were sufficiently established that they could not be ignored. The Federal Employees Health Benefits Program (FEHBP), described in Chapter 5, made choice of plan a central principle. In 1971 Odin Anderson and Joel May of the University of Chicago published a booklet entitled *The Federal Employees Health Benefits Program, 1961–1968; A Model for National Health Insurance?*[1] In 1972 Herman and Anne Somers of Princeton University presented a paper that reviewed existing proposals for national health insurance and also suggested the FEHBP as the basis for a national program.[2] In 1972 and 1973 Scott Fleming, who had represented the Kaiser program in the development of the FEHBP, was serving as Deputy Assistant Secretary in DHEW. As a part of the administration's review of health insurance options, he outlined a proposal that he called Structured Competition in the Private Sector, also modeled on the FEHBP. Unfortunately, this important memorandum did not get the attention it deserved, and the Nixon administration chose a job-centered model as the basis for its National Health Insurance proposal (see Appendix). In 1975 Walter J. McNerney, President of the Blue Cross Association (now Blue Cross–Blue Shield) told the Ways and Means Committee of the House of Representatives that the FEHBP approach was a workable and effective model that could be extended to national health insurance with but few modifications.[3]

In the spring of 1977 President Carter repeated his campaign promise to enact a comprehensive program of national health insurance. The leading proposals at the time all involved large increases in the government's role; none was based on economic competition in the private sector. Because I had become convinced that such competition was a necessary part of any satisfactory plan, I worked through the summer of 1977 as a consultant to HEW Secretary Joseph Califano to convert the previous broad conceptual statements of national health insurance on the FEHBP model into a detailed practical proposal that could actually be implemented. In September 1977 I gave Califano a memorandum proposing Consumer Choice Health Plan (CCHP).[4]

Califano and his associates, however, chose to recommend to President Carter that his administration adopt an approach based on the existing system with increased regulation (see Appendix). In 1979 the proposals of the Carter administration, CCHP, or any other comprehensive proposal appeared to have no chance of enactment in the near future. Still, CCHP remains, in my judgment, the best comprehensive proposal. And it serves as a guide and logical goal for those who favor the concept of a universal system based on fair competition, but want to proceed in smaller steps. (See Chapter 8.)

MAIN IDEAS

Universal Health Insurance Independent of Job Status: Consumer-Centered Rather than Job-Centered Health Insurance[5]

Consumer Choice Health Plan is based on several main ideas. The first is universal health insurance independent of job status. In Chapter 2 I explained how the tax laws contribute to making the employee group the predominant basis for health insurance for people who are neither aged nor poor. Other factors have also contributed to the development of this system. Today's job-centered system of health insurance is largely the by-product of a series of federal actions in the 1940s and 1950s focusing on wage controls, labor relations, and taxes, not on the structure of the health insurance industry. Employer health-benefits contributions were excluded from World War II wage ceilings. In 1948 the National Labor Relations Board ruled health benefits an appropriate subject for collective bargaining. The Internal Revenue Code of 1954 confirmed the exclusion of employer-paid health benefits from the taxable incomes of employees. The consequence of these actions was to tie most people's health insurance to the job of the head of the family. It doesn't have to be that way.

In Chapter 5 I explained how this job-related system works to limit people's choice of health plan and to block competition. It adds enormously to the costs of a new alternative delivery system that is trying to start up.

The link between jobs and health insurance also has other negative consequences. It means that those without employer-provided health insurance often have great difficulty getting health insurance, especially if they have medical problems. People without jobs are considered "an adversely selected group." That is, their expected medical costs are higher than those of people who have jobs. Suppose that a certain number of people leave their jobs and buy health insurance on an individual basis. As time goes by, some of them will get other jobs and drop their individual policies. Others will decide that their health is good, that they are unlikely to need health insurance, and that they can drop their insurance. The people most likely to keep paying their individual premiums, then, are ones who have not gone back to work and who think that they are likely to need their health insurance. By the nature of this selection process, their medical costs will be higher, on the average, than those of employed people in general. Because of the practice of experience rating, these people must pay very high premiums, often for poor benefits, if they can get health insurance at all. Moreover, they are likely to have to pass a medical examination to get insurance, and the costs of treatment of previously existing medical problems are likely to be excluded from coverage.

Thus the link between jobs and health insurance means that people lose their insurance when they lose their jobs, which may be when they need it most. This irony is compounded by the fact that some people must give up their jobs because of poor health. Others lose their health insurance because of the death of the breadwinner on whom they are dependent; others because of divorce or because they have reached the age of majority, but still are not employed.

The job-related system is also the source of many administrative complexities. Some national health insurance proposals attempt to base universal coverage on the employer-provided plans. These proposals would exacerbate the complexities already inherent in today's system. Such proposals assume, implicitly, that everybody is a member of a "typical family" headed by one earner continuously employed at one full-time job. But millions of people do not fit that model. For example, of roughly 20 million manufacturing workers, about 800,000 leave their jobs each month. In the spring of 1977 of 47.5 million families with husband and wife present, about 27.2 million, or 57 percent, had two or more earners. About 4.6 million people held two or more jobs. This helps to explain why, as mentioned earlier, some 34 to 44 million people have duplicate insurance coverage. This is wasteful. It can produce excess insurance costs, with some people collecting twice for the same bill. It can defeat the intended incentives in coinsurance. And it creates a need for "coordination of benefit" rules whereby the overlapping insurers sort out which is to pay what.

People who change jobs are usually forced to change health insurance plans, with gaps in coverage, new starts on annual deductibles, and possible exclusions or waiting periods for preexisting medical conditions. If everybody has an insured fee-for-service health insurance plan with "free choice of doctor," a change in jobs need not mean a change in providers. But in a world of competing alternative delivery systems, the job link adds a new dimension of complexity. People may be forced to change doctors when they change jobs if the new employer does not offer the "limited choice of doctor" plan to which they belonged previously. This may mean new starts on medical records and doctor-patient relationships.

The job–health insurance link adds greatly to administrative complexity in other ways. Each employer negotiates a package with the insurance company, with a special mix of benefits, coinsurance schedules, and provisions concerning cash flow and experience rating. Many of the variations are idiosyncratic and add little or nothing to consumer choice or better health care at less cost. It would make more sense if each insurer offered one or two standard policies to the whole community.

In the job-related system, it has also proved to be very difficult to arrange good health insurance coverage for persons in marginal industries or with seasonal, intermittent, or otherwise unstable employment. Thus low-paid employees, who often need the most protection, get the least.

One of the main foundations of Consumer Choice Health Plan is the principle that every family should have the opportunity to enroll in any health plan active in the area in which it lives and that it should be able to remain continuously enrolled regardless of changes in job status. Moreover, the premium the family pays should reflect the costs of all people cared for by the health plan and should not be higher because one of its members has above-average medical costs or because the co-workers of the breadwinner happen to have greater medical costs.

Equitable Distribution of Public Funds

Another consequence of the tax laws described in Chapter 2 is that the tax subsidies do more for the well-insured well-to-do than for the working poor, who need help more. That is, a well-paid worker with a comprehensive health insurance plan provided by his or her employer may be getting a tax subsidy worth more than $1000 per year. At the same time, an intermittently employed worker without an employer-provided health plan gets no tax subsidy. Moreover, the exclusion of the employer's contribution from the employee's taxable income is worth more to the higher-paid employee, as well as to the employee who chooses a more expensive health plan.

Similarly, Medicare pays more on behalf of beneficiaries with higher incomes than for beneficiaries with lower incomes.[6] Although the benefits are formally the same, regardless of incomes, higher-income people are more likely to live in areas where doctors like to live and hence to be better served. Moreover, they are less likely to be deterred from seeking care by the Medicare coinsurance and deductibles.

The second main idea on which Consumer Choice Health Plan is based is that public funds should be used equitably. Subsidies to people to help them pay for health insurance would be based on the average cost of premiums in their medical-risk category (see below). The subsidies would not vary with income, except in the case of low-income people, who would get more help, based on their financial need.

Reform Through Incentives

The third main idea on which Consumer Choice Health Plan is based is reform of the health care delivery system through incentives. To achieve comprehensive, affordable care of good quality for all, we must change the fundamental structure of the health care financing and delivery system. Instead of today's fragmented system dominated by the cost-increasing incentives of fee for service, I believe that we need a health care economy made up predominantly, though not exclusively, of competing organized systems. In such systems physicians would accept responsibility for providing comprehensive health care services to voluntarily enrolled populations, largely for a per capita payment set in advance in the marketplace or some other form of payment that rewards economy in the use of health care resources.

As we have seen, physicians control the lion's share of health care expenditures. Physicians are by far the best qualified to make the difficult judgments about need and cost effectiveness. Because of the nature of medical care, physician judgment is a far more appropriate basis for resource allocation than are uniform numerical standards. Thus it makes sense for physicians to accept the main responsibility for keeping health care costs within the limits desired by society.

The government cannot reorganize the health care economy by direct action. People would resist such changes involuntarily imposed. And nobody can bring about such a change quickly. But the government can change the underlying economic incentives so that consumers and providers of care can benefit from forming and joining organized systems that use resources wisely. The delivery system would then be forced to reorganize itself in response to consumers who are seeking out and choosing what is in their own best interests. Consumer Choice Health Plan seeks to accomplish this transformation by voluntary changes in a competitive market.

Consumer Choice Health Plan is aimed at correcting today's cost-increasing incentives. It would take money now used to subsidize people's choice of more costly systems of care and use it to raise the floor under the least well covered. It would give consumers an incentive to seek out systems that provide care economically by letting them keep the savings. The government would ensure that people have enough money to enroll in a good plan. But beyond this subsidy level, the economically self-sufficient would be using their own (net after-tax) money, which should motivate them to seek value for it.

Make the Market Work

The fourth main idea of Consumer Choice Health Plan is a positive program on the part of government to make the market work. For example, the government should run or supervise the annual enrollment process to be sure that all persons actually have a choice among all of the competing alternatives. Government should also seek to ensure that people have good information on which to base their choices. An integral part of the program would be a systematic effort to make health-plan choices understandable to consumers. Government would also oversee the rules intended to ensure that competition emphasizes quality of benefits and total costs and not such undesirable practices as preferred-risk selection.

Demonstrated Practical Experience

Finally, Consumer Choice Health Plan's design is based on principles that have actually been applied successfully. Although the concerted application of all the parts of CCHP would be new, each of the parts has been tried on a large scale and found to be practical in application. As noted earlier, CCHP is modeled after the Federal Employees Health Benefits Program, which now serves 10 million people, and similar nonfederal programs, such as the California plan for public employees. CCHP would extend to the whole population and to all qualifying health plans its proven principles of competition, multiple choice, private underwriting and management of health plans, periodic government-supervised open enrollment, and equal rates for all similar enrollees selecting the same plan and benefits.

THE FINANCING SYSTEM

Actuarial Categories and Costs

The amount of government subsidies to individuals to help them buy health insurance would be based on "actuarial cost," the average per capita cost for covered services for persons in each actuarial category. An "actuarial category" is a set of people designated for purposes of premium rating. A good starting point would be a rating structure in widespread use today in which the population under age sixty-five is divided into "individual adults," "individuals plus one dependent" (or couples), and "individuals plus two or more dependents" (or families). For persons sixty-five and over, the population would be divided into categories based on age, sex, location, and other factors determining predicted medical need. Actuarial cost initially would reflect location, because there are large regional differentials in health care costs. The appropriate geographic unit would probably be the state. However, regional differences in real per capita subsidies based on actuarial cost would be phased out over a decade. (Age, sex, and location are the most widely used predictors of medical costs of groups of people. The Medicare program reports data in such categories.)

Actuarial costs for each of these categories would be estimated for a base year at the beginning of the program and would be updated each year by a suitable price index. Subsidies to individuals and families would be set at a fixed percentage of actuarial cost (see below).

For example, the average per capita cost for physician and hospital care in 1978 was about $200 for people under nineteen and about $475 for people nineteen to sixty-four years of age. So actuarial cost for a typical family of four would have been $1350 in that year, if we assume that physician and hospital care are the covered services. A higher or lower amount, based on a more or less extensive list of covered services and on broad political judgments about priorities, might be chosen as the basis for the subsidies. These numbers should be taken as approximations for illustrative purposes. (For technical reasons, I found it easier to do the illustrative examples and cost estimates in terms of individuals rather than the categories mentioned above; I assume that the actual system would use those categories.)

In Consumer Choice Health Plan each health plan would set its own premiums for each actuarial category on the basis of its own costs and its own judgment of what it can charge in a competitive market. Thus persons in actuarial categories having higher costs would pay higher premiums. The government would then alleviate the burden on such people by giving them higher subsidies through tax credits or vouchers.

Although all health plans would be required to accept and care for all persons who signed up with the plan during the open-enrollment period (see below), it would still be important to compensate health plans for serving people with above-average expected medical costs. If health plans were not so compensated, they would have an incentive to find ways to discourage such people from enrolling with them and to encourage the enrollment of low-risk people. For example, a health care plan might recruit an outstanding pediatrics department, to encourage the enrollment of healthy young families, but offer a weak cardiology program, to discourage the enrollment of people with heart problems. That is why health plans should be allowed to charge higher premiums to people in actuarial categories having higher costs. In order to motivate good service to older people in poorer health, the program should make serving them just as attractive financially as serving younger people.

It is possible that experience would show that a more refined set of actuarial categories is desirable. For example, the "three-part structure" described above might be supplemented by special categories for persons aged forty-five to sixty-four. The SAFECO Insurance Company, whose primary care network plan was described in Chapter 4, divides the population it serves in each geographic area into seven actuarial categories based on age and sex. The important thing is that the categories used for premium rating match the categories used for setting subsidies.

This system of premium rating and premium subsidies by actuarial category will not compensate health plans perfectly for serving persons with higher expected medical costs. There would remain some disincentive to enrolling higher-risk persons. However, I believe that such a system can do a good enough job to make the remaining problem of incentives to select preferred risks quite manageable.

Tax Credits

As we saw in Chapter 2, today the health insurance premium contributions of employers and health and welfare funds are excluded from the taxable incomes of employees, and within limits individuals' premium contributions are allowed as itemized deductions. These are, in effect, large tax subsidies toward the purchase of health insurance. In 1979 they cost states and the federal government roughly $14 billion in foregone income and payroll tax revenues.[7]

In CCHP these exclusions and deductions would be replaced by a "refundable tax credit" equal to 60 percent of the family's actuarial cost. A "tax credit" is a flat amount subtracted from the family's tax liability. A "refundable tax credit" means that the family actually gets a cash refund if its credit is greater than its tax liability, not counting the credit. In effect, it is a simple and convenient way for the federal government to transfer money to a taxpayer. The credit would not depend on the family's choice of health plan and, except for poor people, would not depend on income. Employees' tax withholdings would be adjusted, as they are today, to make each taxpayer's total taxes withheld each year approximately equal to the final total tax liability. Employees would not have to wait until the end of the year to receive the tax credit.

Employers and health and welfare funds would continue contributing to employee health insurance under existing agreements, but they would report such contributions as part of total pay on the employees' W-2 forms, and employees would include these amounts as a part of their taxable incomes. The tax credit would offset the additional taxes. The tax credit would be allowed only if the employer and employee had spent that much or more on premiums for a qualified health plan. (See below for an explanation of a "qualified" health plan.) People would not be free to keep the money if they did not join a health plan. Thus this would be a form of compulsory premium contribution through the tax system. The taxpayer would support a claim for the tax credit by stapling to his or her tax return an "H-2" form (like the W-2), a receipt from a qualified health plan stating that the health plan had received premium payments on behalf of the employee from a private source (the employer or the employee). Thus to the ordinary employee, CCHP would appear initially as a very simple change in the way his or her total pay is taxed. For the great majority of people, it would not mean a tax increase, but it would mean an important change in incentives with respect to health insurance purchases.

Consider a typical employee with a family whose employer contributes $1600 per year to the family's health insurance. Under CCHP, his or her personal income tax and Social Security tax would increase roughly $640 because of the inclusion of the $1600 in taxable income (assuming a 40 percent bracket for federal and state income taxes and Social Security taxes combined) and decline by $810 (60 percent of the estimated actuarial cost of $1350) because of the tax credit, for a net saving of $170. (Whether the employee would gain or lose would depend on his or her tax bracket, actuarial category, and previous level of employer-paid benefits.) The importance of the change is that the $810 subsidy would be the same for people with higher and lower incomes (above the low-income line at which special subsidies would begin) and that the subsidy would not increase if the employee chose a more costly health plan.

The choice of 60 percent of actuarial cost as the level for the tax credit is based on a judgment that balances a number of factors. If the tax credit were too low (below 25 percent of actuarial cost), many low-risk employee groups might find it advantageous to form a nonqualified plan and stay out of the system. For the incentives of the system to have their intended effects, most people must find it to their advantage to join qualified plans. Moreoever, a tax credit at least as large as the tax benefit in the present law for middle-income taxpayers would avoid reducing government support for health insurance for that group.

If the tax credit were too high (over 80 percent of actuarial cost), the incentives for health plans to be truly efficient would be weakened. There would be no point in plans' reducing premiums below the tax-credit level. Medicare experience suggests that prepaid group practices can deliver comprehensive health care services for an average of 73 percent of the cost of their fee-for-service counterparts. The tax-credit level should not be above that. Also, if the tax credit were too high, too many consumers would see too little of their own money going into premiums to be motivated to shop for or help form more efficient systems.

A tax credit at 60 percent of actuarial cost would limit the potential for people to manipulate the system to their advantage by taking a minimum-cost "catastrophic expense only" plan when they expected to be healthy and then switching to a comprehensive plan when they anticipated incurring high costs. (See Chapters 1 and 5.) This level approximates the level of subsidy paid by the government in the FEHBP and has worked well. However, other levels could be chosen, depending on the availability of funds. For example, the tax credit could be set at 30 percent initially, with higher levels phased in as revenues permitted.

Vouchers for the Poor

The poor need a higher subsidy to ensure their access to an acceptable plan. CCHP would provide them with a voucher usable only as a premium contribution to the qualified plan of their choice. It should be administered through the cash-assistance welfare system, because that system is already set up to evaluate the incomes and needs of poor people. But the vouchers should be available to all low-income people, not just those presently eligible for welfare. The dollar value of the voucher should be related to family income and should decline gradually with increasing income on a sliding scale that preserves work incentives.

Here is one example. The Carter administration's 1977 welfare-reform proposal would have guaranteed a family of four a minimum cash income of $4200; the cash assistance would be reduced 50 cents for each dollar of earned income until it reached zero at a family income of $8400 (the "cash-assistance break-even" point). Related to this, one could set the health insurance premium voucher at $1350 for a family with a total income, including cash assistance, of $4200 (zero earned income) and phase it down to $810—the tax-credit level for nonpoor families—at a total income of $8400. The result would be a "benefit-reduction rate" (the amount of cash assistance and voucher value lost for each additional dollar earned) of 56 percent, which would not be inconsistent with the goal of preserving work incentives. (People who earn an extra dollar should be allowed to keep a substantial part of it.) If the dollar value of the voucher exceeds the premium for the plan the family chooses, the extra money could be left on deposit to help the family pay for additional health benefits such as dentistry or for any direct medical expenses such as copayments. The voucher system can be designed so that it ties in to the tax system and the unemployment-insurance system without great complexity.

To illustrate how the voucher system would work, suppose that the premium rates in effect for a family in a particular area were $1500 a year for Plan A, $1350 for Plan B, and $1200 for Plan C. If a family of four were totally dependent on welfare, it would receive, using the amounts proposed for 1978 by the Carter administration, a voucher worth $1350 per year for health insurance and cash assistance of $4200 per year. The family could elect Plan C and have $150 per year left over for additional health benefits (such as dentistry, eyeglasses, or to help with any copayments); elect Plan B, in which case the voucher would just equal the premium; or elect Plan A and have to contribute $150 per year out of its cash assistance. If the family's earned income were half way between zero and the "cash-assistance break-even," the voucher would be half way between the $1350 available to families with no earned income and the $810 available to nonpoor families, or $1080. These numbers are illustrative; the actual voucher level might be different, depending on such factors as political judgments and regional cost levels. I would expect competition to keep the difference in premiums among the plans within fairly narrow limits, so that low-income families would not be limited in their effective choices to the least costly plans.

Medicare

Medicare would be retained for the aged, disabled, and victims of chronic kidney failure. But it would be reformed in a very fundamental way, in two stages.

The first step would be a "freedom-of-choice" provision. Today, the Medicare program keeps track of the per capita costs to Medicare for people in various categories defined mainly by age, sex, and location. For example, the Health Care Financing Administration can state the average per capita cost to Medicare for males aged sixty-five to seventy in Seattle in 1975. Statistical methods have been developed, using indices of recent price changes, to project from actual past expenses to estimates of what an average person in each category will cost next year. This amount is called the "adjusted average per capita cost" for people in that category. The first step of reform would permit beneficiaries to direct that an amount equal to their adjusted average per capita cost be paid, as a premium contribution, to the qualified health plan of their choice. (For this amount, the health plan would have to provide at least the same level of benefits as are provided by the Medicare program.)

The point of this change would be to permit beneficiaries to realize for themselves the benefits of joining an economical alternative delivery system, in the form of a reduced premium, or reduced (or eliminated) coinsurance and deductibles, or a more extensive list of covered services. As a result of such a change, Medicare would no longer pay more on behalf of those who choose more costly providers.

For example, as I explained in Chapter 5, in 1970 Medicare paid $202 per capita on behalf of beneficiaries cared for by Group Health Cooperative of Puget Sound, but paid $356 on behalf of similar beneficiaries in the same area who got their care from the fee-for-service sector. Nevertheless, as far as Medicare was concerned, the Group Health members were liable for the same deductibles and coinsurance and subject to the same limitations on covered hospital days as their counterparts who chose fee for service. They received no reward from Medicare for choosing a less costly system. The government kept all the savings. If Consumer Choice Health Plan had been in effect, they would have been allowed to designate that $356 be paid by Medicare as a premium contribution on their behalf to Group Health Cooperative or another qualified health plan. Group Health would have been able to pass on the extra $154 to the beneficiaries by reducing or eliminating coinsurance or deductibles, by removing the limitation on hospital days covered, by increasing the scope of benefits to include health care expenses not otherwise covered by Medicare, or by reducing any supplemental premium. In a competitive situation, Group Health would have to pass on such savings to beneficiaries in order to attract them to join.

However, this reform would be only an interim step. It would leave the costs of the Medicare program tied to the cost of providers working under the cost-increasing incentives of cost reimbursement and fee for service. The "adjusted average per capita cost" factors are defined on the basis of the costs of beneficiaries served by the fee-for-service sector, including the costs of the most costly providers. In fact, after a time, as substantial numbers of beneficiaries shifted out of the fee-for-service sector, the "freedom-of-choice" provision would tend to accelerate the rate of increase in average fee-for-service costs in two ways. The first providers to switch to alternative delivery systems are likely to be the most economical, leaving the less economical in the fee-for-service sector. Also, as noted in Chapters 3 and 4, some alternative delivery systems, such as prepaid group practices, care for their members with fewer doctors and hospital beds per capita than does the fee-for-service sector. Thus as these alternative delivery systems gain increased membership, more doctors and hospital beds per capita are left in the fee-for-service sector. And, as explained in Chapter 2, this will mean higher per capita costs in the fee-for-service sector.

Therefore, a second stage of reform is needed in which the subsidies paid by government are disconnected from the costs of the fee-for-service sector. In this stage all new Medicare beneficiaries, as of a certain date, would be covered by a new system in which their subsidies would be fixed in real terms, and they would be given an annual choice of all of the qualified health plans operating in their area. These subsidies would be equal to the "adjusted average per capita cost" factors, for people in each category, in the first year of the program. The subsidies in subsequent years would increase in proportion to a suitable price index.

All previously covered Medicare beneficiaries who wanted to choose private qualified health plans could choose to receive these fixed premium contributions in lieu of their regular Medicare coverage. Previously covered beneficiaries who wanted to remain on the old system of fee for service and cost reimbursement would be free to do so. As the years went by, the population cared for under the old Medicare system would diminish, and eventually the new system would completely replace the old one. The government's per capita expense would be stabilized in real terms (net of inflation), because its per capita subsidies (or premium contributions) would be fixed in real terms.

In 1978 about 7.7 million poor, blind, and disabled aged persons received Medicaid supplements to assist with costs not covered by Medicare. (Medicare pays about 71 percent of hospital costs and 55 percent of physician costs for aged beneficiaries.) Under CCHP, these supplements for acute care would be replaced by a voucher similar to that for the nonaged poor. This substitution would ensure the ability of the Medicare beneficiary with a low income to pay the premiums for a policy to supplement Medicare. In 1978 the average per capita hospital and physician costs for the aged, not covered by Medicare, were about $385. This would be an appropriate value for the full voucher to supplement Medicare.

Regional Differences

There is a serious problem of regional differentials in health care spending. For example, in 1977 hospital expenditures per capita for all residents were $137 in Wyoming and $349 in Massachusetts—57 and 146 percent, respectively—of the national average. A uniform national system of subsidies set on the basis of average cost would mean hardship in high-cost areas and overly generous subsidies in low-cost areas. Yet it would be difficult to defend a permanent state of inequality. Why should states whose health care providers did a poor job of controlling costs get a permanent subsidy at the expense of those states whose providers did a good job?

There are various ways this could be handled in the context of CCHP, and there would doubtless be a considerable amount of negotiation and political compromise in the eventual resolution of the problem. One good way would be to adjust the subsidies (tax credits and vouchers) to reflect state-by-state relative differences in health care costs in the first year, but to phase out the differences on a straight-line basis over a ten-year period. Thus citizens in a state with costs 50 percent above the national average would get a tax credit 50 percent above the national average in the first year, but equal to the national average in the tenth year. This would give providers time to adapt. Hospitals in overbedded areas could be reduced in size or converted to other uses. New physicians would consider the changing pattern of subsidies in their decisions as to where to locate.

CREATING A SOCIALLY DESIRABLE COMPETITION: CRITERIA FOR QUALIFIED HEALTH PLANS

To qualify to receive tax credits, vouchers, or Medicare payments, a health plan would have to operate according to a set of rules intended to create a fair and socially desirable competition based on quality and economy. The essential ideas are described on the following pages.

Open Enrollment

Each plan would be required to participate in an annual government-supervised open enrollment in which it would have to accept all eligible persons choosing to join it, without regard to age, sex, race, religion, national origin, or prior health conditions. Once a year, every family would receive an informative booklet, published by the CCHP administrative agency, giving an understandable presentation of the costs, covered services, service locations, and participating providers of each qualified health plan in the area. Each family would make a selection for the coming year through an employer, welfare office, or local office of the administrative agency.

Annual open enrollment would greatly enhance competition by giving each person a choice from among competing plans, and it would ensure that every person could enroll in a qualified plan.

The enrollment process should be run by a government agency, for several reasons. An impartial agency is needed to ensure that the information presented is complete, balanced, and fair. Such an agency is needed to ensure that every eligible person is truly given an opportunity to enroll in the plan of his or her choice. Otherwise, health plans might be able to make it difficult for higher-risk persons to join. A government-run enrollment would obviate the need for each health plan to have its own sales personnel and promotional materials. This would reduce cost and help prevent the kind of marketing abuses associated with the scandal of southern California prepaid health plans in the early 1970s (see Chapter 4). The procedures would be modeled after the Federal Employees program and other similar public- and private-sector multiple-choice plans.

Community Rating

A qualified plan would be required to charge the same premium to all persons in the same actuarial category enrolled for the same benefits in the same area. This practice is called "community rating." The reasons for it were explained in Chapter 5. Community rating is fundamental to any system of universal coverage based on fair competition. If it were not required, health plans could charge high premiums to high-risk persons, in effect making health insurance unaffordable to those who need it most.

I doubt that we will ever be able to make affordable health insurance available to the unemployed and to others cut off from membership in employee groups, without a system of community rating. The fact that the prototype HMOs have used community rating for decades shows that it is entirely feasible.

Basic Health Services

A qualified health plan would be required to cover, at a minimum, the list of services called "basic health services" in the HMO Act of 1973 (as amended). That list includes physician services, inpatient and outpatient hospital services, emergency health services, short-term outpatient mental health services (up to twenty visits), treatment and referral for drug and alcohol abuse, laboratory, and X-ray, home health services, and certain preventive health services. It might make sense to start the program with a less costly list. The point is not that there is anything sacred about this particular list of services, but that we need some agreed on, uniform definition of "all the care you need" that is applicable to all health plans. This coverage might be subject to substantial copayments (such as $5 per doctor visit) and deductibles, and additional benefits could be offered.

A list of basic health services is needed as a common yardstick, for several reasons. Today, the covered benefits of health plans are often difficult to understand and compare. There are tricky exclusions and limits on coverage; indeed, doctors refer to some as "swiss cheese policies." Such policies are often designed to protect the insurer and to make price comparisons difficult. Consumers can understand copayments and deductibles and make reasonable judgments about quality and accessibility of services. But the effort and cost to become well informed about the significance of many "fine print" exclusions can be very great. The requirement to cover basic health services would standardize a lot of fine print. All policies could then be described in terms of basic health services plus a manageable number of additional benefits. This would help to focus competition on the quality and accessibility of services and price. Price comparisons would be easier and more meaningful, and consumers would be protected from misleading exclusions of important services.

Premium Rating by Market Area

Consumer Choice Health Plan would be organized on the basis of market areas, usually states, but in a few cases two or three economic zones in a state. Qualified plans would be required to set their community rates on the basis of these market areas, so that the premiums in each area would reflect the costs in that area. Today, citizens in low-cost areas are paying taxes and premiums to subsidize excess hospitalization in high-cost areas. Such subsidies reduce the incentive for economical behavior.

Low Option

Qualified plans would be required to offer a "low-option" plan limited to basic health services. They could also offer one or more higher-option plans. The main purpose of this requirement would be to prevent plans from limiting membership to the well-to-do by offering only plans with costly supplemental benefits. It would also help to sharpen price competition by requiring all plans to quote prices for one common package of covered services.

"Catastrophic Expense Protection"

Qualified plans must publish a clearly stated annual limit on family out-of-pocket outlays for covered services. A suitable limit would be $1500. Out-of-pocket outlays include deductibles, copayments, and, in the case of indemnity insurance plans, any differences between indemnity payments and the actual cost of covered services. Beyond the limit, the health plan must pay for all of the costs of covered services. This requirement would help ensure that health plans do not compete by offering inadequate benefits that would leave the seriously ill uninsured or dependent on the public sector. It would provide full protection against catastrophic medical expenses and prevent "medical bankruptcies."

Copayments and deductibles may play a useful role in helping to control consumer-initiated use of services. The appropriate role for copayments and deductibles is a controversial topic. Some people consider them essential to discourage inappropriate use of services. Others oppose them strongly. Whatever can be said for their value in discouraging unnecessary doctor office visits, copayments or coinsurance are not likely to change anything at all when the patient is seriously ill and has been in the hospital several days. Then it is the doctor who is making the key cost-generating decisions. I see no value in requiring the patient to pay a part of the bill in such circumstances. Assuming the typical 20 or 25 percent coinsurance rate, a $1500 limit on the family's out-of-pocket outlays means that the health plan must pay all costs after the family has had gross medical expenses of some $6000 or $7500. When expenses are that large, the patient is likely to be quite ill and not susceptible to the economic incentives of coinsurance. Health plans would be free to set their own deductibles and copayments within this limit.

Qualified plans would be permitted to require that their members obtain all of their covered benefits from participating providers with whom they have made agreements concerning fees and utilization controls (except for emergency treatment). Indeed, the pressure of economic competition would gradually force health plans to make such agreements. But if a plan did not have an agreement with a participating provider in a needed specialty, it would nevertheless have to pay the cost and "hold the consumer harmless" within the agreed cost-sharing limits.

Information Disclosure

A program to provide meaningful, useful information on the features and merits of alternative health plans would be an essential part of CCHP and a major departure from present practice. To aid consumer choice, each plan would be required to publish total per capita costs, including premiums and out-of-pocket costs. The government administrative agency would have authority to review and approve promotional materials (for accuracy and balance), including information presented in the booklet available to all eligible persons at enrollment. The administrative agency would also have authority to review and approve contract language so that all options offered would either conform to a standard contract or be described by a standard contract and a manageable number of additions and exclusions. The purpose of this would be to publish health plan information in a format understandable to consumers and that facilitates direct comparison among plans without forcing the consumer to master and compare a lot of fine print. Uniform financial disclosure would be required—comparable to what the Securities and Exchange Commission requires of public companies. Data on patterns of utilization and availability and accessibility of services would be required, as is required of health maintenance organizations.

Health Plan Identification Card

Every qualified plan would issue each member a card that would inform providers of a person's health plan membership and that would serve as a credit card for covered services for eligible providers. This would virtually eliminate questions of payment at the provider's office, and it would put the burden of credit and collection on the health plan rather than on the individual provider, for health plans are better equipped to handle financial matters. Revolving credit at regulated interest rates would ease the cash-flow problem for persons facing large out-of-pocket payments.

FEDERAL-STATE ROLES IN FINANCING AND ADMINISTRATION

CCHP is compatible with many possible ways of splitting federal and state financing and administrative responsibilities. The choice must be considered in the context of federal-state sharing of financial burdens in general (of which acute medical-care financing is only one piece), and it must rest largely on political judgments. Because states are potentially important factors in health facilities planning and cost controls, the federal government should not pay more on behalf of states that have higher per capita health care costs in such a way as to weaken their incentive to control costs. CCHP could be administered entirely by the federal government or by the states under federal standards.

SPECIAL CATEGORIES—DEFENSE DEPARTMENT, VETERANS, INDIANS, MIGRANTS, THE UNDERWORLD, ILLEGAL ALIENS, NONENROLLERS, OTHERS

Beneficiaries of Public Direct-Care Systems

More than 9 million persons are eligible for medical care through the Military Health Services System. Eligibles include about 2.1 million active-duty military personnel and about 7 million civilians, including dependents of active-duty personnel, retired military and their dependents, and survivors. The Civilian Health and Medical Program of the Uniformed Services (CHAMPUS) is a financing program that provides for the payment of health services bills incurred in the civilian sector by nonactive-duty eligibles. Total Defense Department medical and health outlays for 1978 were budgeted at about $3.9 billion, of which about $2.6 billion was for direct hospital and medical services, whereas CHAMPUS accounted for $654 million.

Roughly 26 million veterans are eligible for Veterans Administration (VA) health care benefits, although many get their care through other sources. In 1978 the VA budget provided for inpatient care for 1.4 million veterans and 18.2 million outpatient medical and dental visits. The VA health budget was $5.1 billion, of which $4.3 billion was for hospital and medical services. The federal government also budgeted $472 million, including $227 for hospital and medical services, for health care for 564,000 American Indians. Many of these people also receive tax-subsidized, employer-paid insurance through their civilian employers. Thus we have double tax subsidies, and it is impossible to estimate the adjusted per capita costs of these public systems, because the eligibles do not get all their care in one system.

In CCHP each person eligible for one of these systems of care would be required to make a choice (which could be revised periodically); he or she might elect either the tax credit or continued care through the government system, but not both. This would bring about a desirable alignment between health care systems and the defined populations they serve. That is, each year, each person would belong to one or another system. That system would then be responsible for planning resources for his or her care. The element of choice would also begin to put some competitive pressure on the government direct-care systems.

Migrants, Derelicts, the Underworld, Illegal Aliens, Nonenrollers, Others

What should be done about migrant workers, incompetents, persons in illegal occupations who do not want to sign up for tax credits or vouchers, illegal aliens, and persons who, though eligible, for one reason or another do not enroll in a health plan? Any attempt to achieve universal coverage must deal with the special problems of these people. CCHP by itself does not "solve" these problems, any more than any other national health insurance proposal would. CCHP does create a framework that is helpful in addressing some of these problems, but, generally speaking, special programs are required for special problems.

Under any scheme, there will be a need for a system of public providers of last resort. Such public systems could "enroll" nonenrolled persons as they need care and claim the funds provided by their unused tax credits or vouchers.

Migrant workers will need a system designed to cope with their special problems. Again, CCHP's vouchers could provide the vehicle to finance such a system.

As for the problem of eligibles who fail to enroll, welfare recipients could be counseled or required to choose a plan as part of the process of registering to receive assistance. Special rules could be worked out for other nonenrolled eligibles. For example, a system similar to one that has been used in the private sector for union members in dual-choice plans who failed to make an election at enrollment time or when they became eligible could be used. The revenues (tax credit or voucher) attributable to those who have not enrolled, in each state, could be divided among the qualified health plans in proportion to their membership or to the number of previously unenrolled who were enrolled by each plan in the previous year. Then when an unenrolled person became sick and sought service, he would be enrolled in the plan of his choice. The divided revenues thus serve as a sort of "commitment fee" to the plans, indemnifying them for the risk entailed in the obligation to enroll previously unenrolled people at the time when they need medical care. Back premium payments might be required in order to make sure that nobody finds it financially advantageous not to enroll in a health plan.

It is important, when designing a system to serve 95 percent of Americans, not to distort it seriously because of the special problems of the other 5 percent.

TRANSITION

The enactment of CCHP would cause no sudden wrenching upheaval in medical care delivery or financing. There would be a transition period, during which health plans intending to qualify would prepare for the first open enrollment. To many plans, this would be a familiar procedure because they already participate in a multiple-choice system. Some insurance companies would seek to obtain signed participation agreements with physicians similar to those already used by Blue Shield. Such agreements would cover fees and cost controls. Some insurance companies would seek to sign up physicians to participate in primary care networks and other alternative delivery systems. Physician groups would doubtless accelerate efforts already under way to form individual practice associations. Various groups would seek to form prepaid group practices. In all probability, Blue Cross-Blue Shield would offer a traditional insured "service-benefit plan" in each market area.

Some physicians would sign agreements to participate in more than one plan. Some would decide to devote their efforts to one plan. Some would decide that the demand for their services was such that they would not need to sign any agreements, although that stance might become economically disadvantageous quite soon. In the first few years of CCHP, most physicians would continue to practice in their same offices and hospitals and to care for the same patients as before.

Gradually, however, competitive economic pressures would have their effect. People would gradually change to more economical health plans. Less economical health plans would have to find more effective cost controls. Newly trained physicians in specialties in excess supply in a given area would find no health plans interested in contracting with them, and they would have to look for work in areas where their services were needed. Primary-care physicians would assume more of the responsibility for the total costs of care for their patients, and specialists whose costs were judged by such primary-care physicians to be excessive would find themselves obliged to negotiate lower fees in order to retain their referrals. Individual practice associations would tighten utilization controls and more carefully balance the specialty mix of their participating physicians to the needs of their enrolled populations. Prepaid group practices would continue to grow.

In short, the competitive market would generate cost controls, but they would be private market controls based on individual and group judgments about cost versus value received, not public controls based on arbitrary uniform standards insensitive to the quality or value of the services and to individual preferences.

PUBLIC POLICY TOWARD DELIVERY-SYSTEM REFORM

CCHP would create a competitive economy whose rules were fair to economical alternative delivery systems. It would correct the biases against them that exist today in the tax laws, Medicare, Medicaid, employer-employee financing arrangements and elsewhere, and it would give them the opportunity to reach their entire potential markets through the government-run open enrollment. It would allow them to pass on to consumers the full benefit of their savings.

But CCHP would not in itself create new alternative delivery systems. If such systems are to come into being, many local efforts to organize them will be required. Such initiatives might be led, as they have been in the past and are being today, by employers, unions, universities, consumer cooperatives, foundations, insurance companies, physician groups, hospitals, and local governments. If additional public policies to encourage such efforts prove to be needed, they should be the subject of separate legislation.

I do not place much confidence in proposals for special grants and other subsidies for HMOs. Experience with the HMO Act shows that such subsidies come at an extremely high price. The HMO Act promised large grants and loans to HMOs, on the basis of which many costly restrictions were justified, burdens that were not placed equally on their competitors. The financial help actually delivered fell far below the amounts originally authorized. Given a truly fair market test, as proposed in CCHP, health plans demonstrating the economic superiority of many existing HMOs will prosper without help. Even the investment capital needed for startup will be far easier to raise if people can be confident that the basic economic ground rules will allow an efficient system to compete successfully.

An antitrust strategy specifically designed for the peculiar economics of the health care industry is needed and is evolving. Ordinary antitrust theory, developed for other industries, does not fit very well in health care. It is easy to imagine some noncompetitive outcomes under Consumer Choice Health Plan. For example, a county medical society might form an individual practice association and use it as a price-fixing arrangement, keeping out would-be competing physicians by controlling hospital privileges. Or, a market might continue to be dominated by several "free-choice-of-doctor" plans, all paying the same providers the same fees and costs, thus precluding real economic competition among doctors.

However, the Federal Trade Commission has substantially upgraded its expertise in health services and has been achieving gains in applying antitrust principles to this field. For example, the FTC staff has recommended that physician organizations be required to divest themselves of control of Blue Shield plans. The Ohio State Medical Society has been forced to give up ownership of Ohio Blue Shield. Medical-society control of individual practice associations, with its obvious monopolistic potential, is under similar challenge. The FTC is watching for boycotts, denials of staff privileges, and other practices that restrain competition and has obtained consent decrees to stop them. The medical profession is going to have to live by the rules of competition accepted by American business in general.

COSTS AND THE FEDERAL BUDGET

Before considering estimates of the costs of any universal health insurance proposal, it is important to recognize the inherent limitations in the estimating methods. Costs are estimated by multiplying recent prices of services by recent per capita rates of use of services and by the size of the covered population. To that is added an estimate of "induced demand," the short-term increase in demand attributable to improved insurance coverage. The calculation must use "best guess" assumptions about induced demand because there is no firmly based estimate of it.

Another problem that seriously compounds the difficulty the ordinary citizen faces in trying to understand national health insurance cost estimates is the recent popularity of what is known as "off-budget financing." Because increases in taxes and federal spending are unpopular, some political leaders have sought ways of financing health insurance that are not called taxes and government spending. Thus the health insurance plan favored by the Carter administration would be paid for by "required health insurance premiums" (see Appendix). And Senator Kennedy's 1979 proposal would be financed by an "earnings-based premium." Some people are likely to use the word "taxes" to describe these compulsory payments, just as the Internal Revenue Service and the federal budget use the phrase "payroll taxes" for what the Social Security Administration likes to refer to as "contributions."

But the most important difficulty in estimating the costs of any national health insurance proposal is that the methods used for producing estimates totally lack any scientific basis for forecasting the long-term effect of the incentives created by that proposal on unit costs, use of services, and standards of care. Hence the estimators are forced to make assumptions with very little but judgment to go on. The history of programs such as Medicare has been one of consistent large underestimation in the long run. In 1965 the 1975 costs of Medicare hospital insurance were projected at $4.3 billion; the actual was about $11.7 billion. Deflate this for the 71 percent increase in general price levels, and one still gets about a 60 percent overrun. There was a similar history in the renal-dialysis program. But the problem is potentially far more serious in a national health insurance program because the size and impact of the program are larger. The key factor determining the total costs in the long run is the effect of the incentives created on unit costs, use of services, and standards of medical care.

The effects of a lack of reliable estimating methods are compounded by the incentives and optimism of proponents of social-insurance programs. Few, if any, people may be seriously interested in realistic estimates when the program is under consideration. What reward is there for realism?

The costs of a program to the government will depend in a major way on whether the system makes them controllable or open-ended and uncontrollable. An important feature of CCHP is that in it, costs to the federal government are controllable and can therefore be estimated with far greater reliability than can the costs of an open-ended third-party reimbursement system.

The costs will depend on the particular services that are covered and the amount of the tax credits and vouchers. Here are some illustrative examples, using 1978 dollars.

Assume that actuarial cost is $200 for a person under nineteen years of age and $475 for persons nineteen to sixty-four. Actuarial cost on the same basis (that is, per capita spending for physicians and hospital services) for a Medicare beneficiary was about $1150. On the average, Medicare pays about 67 percent of this amount. Therefore, a low-income Medicare beneficiary needing 100 percent public support would need a voucher worth $380 in addition to the $770 Medicare would contribute for a person who is not poor.

Now, assume that the tax credit for families that are neither aged nor poor is set at 60 percent of actuarial cost. Let the voucher for a poor family with no income other than cash assistance be 100 percent of actuarial cost. Let the voucher's value be reduced 12 cents for each dollar of family income, including cash assistance, above the income guarantee level (above $4200 for a family of four), until it reaches the amount available to the nonpoor. The total annual cost to the federal budget for these tax credits and vouchers, including the supplemental vouchers for poor Medicare beneficiaries, would be $46.2 billion. (This figure does not include the costs of the existing Medicare program, which are assumed to continue unchanged in the short run.)

Offset against the tax credits and vouchers would be the extra revenues gained from the proposed changes in the federal tax laws (eliminating the exclusion of employer contributions to employee health insurance from the employee's income subject to federal income and Social Security taxes) worth $10.1 billion, federal Medicaid of $11.8 billion, and other programs of $1.9 billion that would be replaced by the tax credits and vouchers, for a total of $23.8 billion. (The states would be relieved of Medicaid acute-care costs, but would pay for all costs of long-term care; this revision would maintain approximately the present federal-state division of costs.) Thus the net additional cost to the federal budget for the full Consumer Choice Health Plan proposal would be about $22.4 billion in 1978 dollars. Initially, total national health care spending would be unchanged, but the federal contribution would be increased.

Alternatively, as the low-cost start of a program to phase in Consumer Choice Health Plan, let the tax credit for the nonpoor be set at 30 percent of actuarial cost. Let the voucher for the poor be 100 percent of actuarial cost for a family at the same income-guarantee level. Let the voucher's value be reduced 20 cents for each dollar of family income (including cash assistance) above that, until it reached the amount available to the nonpoor. The total cost to the federal budget for these tax credits and vouchers would be $26.9 billion. The net cost to the federal budget, after subtraction of the above-mentioned offsets, would be $3.1 billion.

From a fiscal point of view, CCHP would make the government's contribution to personal health services a "controllable" expenditure that could be set at a level in balance with other priorities, instead of today's open-ended commitments through the third-party intermediary, fee-for-service, cost-reimbursement system. Moreover, in CCHP those who wanted more health services would have the option of using their own net after-tax income to buy them, resulting in less pressure on the Congress than there would be if all the costs were paid by the federal government.

Most important, by establishing strong incentives for cost effectiveness, CCHP promises in the long run to reduce total national health care costs to levels considerably below what they otherwise would be.

I did not submit a proposal for how to pay for the $22.4 billion to implement CCHP at the higher level. Because our income tax system takes an increasing percentage of incomes as incomes rise, inflation pushes most people into higher tax brackets each year even if dollar incomes increase only in proportion to the cost of living. Therefore, from time to time, a tax cut is needed in any case. When I proposed CCHP, I suggested that the next tax cut could be made in the form of refundable tax credits for health insurance. Other ways of financing the program would have to be evaluated in the total context of federal general-revenue collection.

To some people, national health insurance is primarily a means for redistributing income. They pay a great deal of attention to the sources of revenue and tend to ignore the impact of their proposals on the structure of the health services industry. From my point of view, the impact of the national health care financing system on the structure of the industry is of the first order of importance. If we can, through appropriate incentives, create an efficient economical health services industry, the question of how to pay for it will become a great deal easier to answer.

CCHP: SOME ISSUES AND ANSWERS

Speed of Reorganization

One of the main criticisms of CCHP by those who favor the regulatory approach is that we cannot wait for reorganization of the delivery system to get costs under control. This argument is based on the premise that direct regulatory approaches can produce results quickly—a premise refuted by the evidence summarized in Chapter 6. A judgment in favor of the competitive market approach must be based, in part, on a realistic appraisal of the alternatives. Reorganization of health services will take a long time, a decade or more before half of the population is served by some kind of organized system with incentives for economy, even under the most favorable conditions. The reasons for this were explained at the end of Chapter 5.

However, the enactment of Consumer Choice Health Plan would accelerate the process of reorganization to a speed considerably faster than the pace of change we have observed to date. For one thing, every family would have a multiple choice of health plan on an economically fair basis, not just the minority that has it today. The loophole of open-ended third-party financing of the fee-for-service sector would be closed. Providers would recognize this and hasten to form or join alternative delivery systems. The growing supply of physicians would accelerate this. Moreover, the costs for a new health plan to enter the market would be reduced greatly from today's high level. Instead of having to meet the requirements of each of hundreds of employers, before they can be offered to most families, new health plans would have to meet only the qualification requirements of the CCHP administrative agency before being offered to all families in their market area.

"Consumer Choice"

Proposals to rely on consumer choice to guide the health services system are invariably subjected to the attack that consumers are incapable of making intelligent choices in health care matters. So it seems worthwhile to make it clear exactly what is being assumed. Admittedly, there is a great deal of ignorance and uncertainty regarding health insurance and care; that is true for physicians and civil servants as well as for ordinary consumers. CCHP does not assume that the ordinary consumer is a perfect judge of what is in his or her own best interest. Consumers may be ignorant, biased, and vulnerable to deception. CCHP merely assumes that when it comes to choosing a health plan, the ordinary consumer is the best judge of what is in his or her own best interest. For a competitive market system to produce good results, it is not necessary that every consumer be perfectly informed and economically rational. Markets can be policed by a minority of well-informed cost-conscious consumers. And we are seeking merely a good and workable solution, not some theoretical optimum. CCHP would provide consumers with substantially better information than they get now and much stronger incentives to use it. If there were a demand for it, much could be done to organize better consumer information.

In any case, the key factor is the incentive that CCHP gives to providers. Provider systems would have to look to satisfied consumers rather than to the government for their revenues. In CCHP above the tax credit/voucher level, consumers would be working with their own money, not somebody else's.

If we can agree, through the political process, that some choices are unwise or antisocial, such as not buying catastrophic expense protection, we can make them ineligible for subsidies. That we take some choices out of the marketplace does not mean that we have to take the entire system out of the market.

Presumably every national health care financing system under consideration would allow each consumer a choice of physician and free choice of whether or not to accept recommended medical treatment—decisions that would be aided by technical knowledge. What distinguishes CCHP from the others is that it seeks to give consumers a choice from among alternative systems for organizing and financing care and to allow them to benefit from their economizing choices. The relevant factors in such a choice are less technical and easier to judge. The issue, then, is whether consumers can be trusted to choose wisely when it comes to picking health plans—some of which cost less than others. Experience with multiple-choice systems, summarized in Chapter 5, shows that consumers are capable of making such choices satisfactorily.

Part of the "consumer-choice" issue is resistance to the idea of letting the poor, because of their poverty, choose a less costly health plan that might not meet their medical needs. There is appearance of a conflict here with the principle of CCHP that people must be allowed to benefit from their economizing choices. The problem can be resolved in CCHP by setting the premium vouchers (usable only for health care) at a high enough level to ensure access to a plan with adequate benefits—always letting plans that do a better job attract members by offering more benefits.

Critics of the consumer-choice position usually are not very explicit about whom they consider to be better qualified than the average American to choose a health plan for him- or herself. In reality the alternative to a consumer-choice system is a provider-dominated system.

Fairness to the Poor

CCHP uses the most effective way to redistribute purchasing power for medical care—that is, directly. It takes money from taxpayers and pays it to lower-income people in the form of tax credits and vouchers. By this method, the amount of redistribution is clearly visible, and one can be sure that the money reaches its intended target. CCHP can thus be used to bring about whatever income redistribution for medical care purchases the political process will support. By contrast, third-party insurance systems are an exceedingly ineffective way to redistribute income. Medicare pays more on behalf of rich than of poor. In a bureaucratic system individuals and organized groups who are forceful and skillful at getting their way come out ahead.

Would CCHP perpetuate a two-class system of care for rich and poor? The question should be judged realistically in terms of where we are today, in which direction CCHP would move us, and where we are likely to go as a society. CCHP focuses on raising the quality of care available to the poor by ensuring that they have the money (through vouchers) and the access (through the government-run open enrollment) to the same health plans that serve middle-income people. Competition is likely to keep the cost of many of these plans within reach for many low-income people. Moreover, unlike the present tax law, CCHP would require the well-to-do to pay the extra cost of more expensive health plans out of their own after-tax incomes. Thus CCHP would be a large step toward equalizing health care purchasing power, without enforcing absolute equality. I believe that it would be foolish to reject CCHP on the grounds that it does not reach a hypothetical egalitarian ideal that has never been attained in any society and is not likely to be attained under any program.

Underserved Rural Areas

CCHP would not "solve" the problem of underserved areas, but it would help. It would ensure medical purchasing power for people in rural areas, many of whom have low incomes. It would end the open-ended tax subsidy to the well-served areas, and it would put financial pressure on physician-location decisions.

The best way to provide good care in rural areas is through organized systems that can provide outreach services and that can provide financial and professional support to physicians working in such areas. For example, Kaiser-Permanente operates remote outposts in Hawaii, including a single-physician clinic on the northern shore of Oahu. Though far from the main medical center, this doctor can easily consult with his specialist partners by telephone and can refer patients if necessary. For a physician facing the choice of where to practice, the prospect of a rural practice can be much more attractive if he or she can be affiliated with a larger group.

"WHAT'S IN IT FOR ME?"

CCHP's design principles are equity, practicality, and rational economics. CCHP was developed with an appreciaton of the broad political realities, a recognition of the need to do something about health care costs, and awareness of the public's growing disenchantment with government regulation. Although Consumer Choice Health Plan may not be the first choice of any particular group, it might, like the Federal Employees Health Benefits Program, well be an acceptable "second best" for many. The answer to the question "What's in it for me?" depends on the alternative. Although many will compare CCHP to the status quo, I believe that the present size and rate of increase in health care costs make the status quo untenable. The real alternative to a plan like CCHP, based on incentives and competition, is a plan based on tight, detailed government control of prices, capacity, and use of services.

Compared with the status quo, economic competition would lead to some loss of income and autonomy for doctors. For example, in a CCHP world doctors would have less freedom to set up practice wherever they pleased. The job market for doctors would look more like the job market for other professionals. Doctors would be free to choose from available alternatives, but the available alternatives would be more closely related to the needs of the people being cared for. But compared with the inevitable economic controls that will come in the absence of effective competition, CCHP offers the medical profession the surest basis for maintaining its autonomy. Such government controls would inevitably be based on arbitrary numerical standards applied across the board without respect for individual preferences or quality. They would involve increasing paperwork of a frustrating and unproductive kind. Medicare regulations have given a taste of what is in store down that road. The politicizing of the negotiating process over physician fees would inevitably be damaging and unpalatable.

By contrast, in an effective system of economic competition, such as that proposed in CCHP, medical care costs could be controlled by the judgment of physicians. Individual preferences would be respected. For this system to work, physicians would have to accept responsibility for managing the total health care costs of their enrolled population groups. Acceptance of such a role would enhance the social contribution and recognition of the profession.

For hospital administrators, CCHP would mean a drop in demand for hospital services and an economic environment similar to that faced by other managers. There would be a transition period, during which excess capacity would be closed or converted to other uses. Some existing hospital facilities would be converted to outpatient care, others to long-term care. But CCHP would mean relief from many burdensome and frustrating government regulations. Today, hospital administrators are placed in a very uncomfortable situation between the open-ended demands created by third-party financing of the fee-for-service system on the one hand and government spending limits on the other. In the system created by CCHP, hospital administrators would set their prices in negotiation with informed cost-conscious buyers who could make judgments about local conditions. Providers would succeed by offering better services at lower costs. The opportunity to do that ought to yield more job satisfaction to providers than they get from the struggle to understand and beat complex government regulations.

For health insurance companies, the status quo is not very promising. Today's group insurance business is not very profitable, and it is giving way to claims-processing services. CCHP would mean a fundamental change in the basis of the business. Pure financial intermediation would be unlikely to survive on a large scale. Insurance companies would have to get involved in organizing, managing, financing, and marketing health plans, something for which their experience should give them a good head start. There would be considerably more opportunities for substantial social contribution in this kind of business than in the traditional insurance business, and it is likely to be more profitable.

For workers, CCHP offers an expanded range of choice and improved efficiency and reduced cost through competition. It also would mean ensured continuity of coverage in the face of job changes or unemployment. Since employer contributions to health insurance really come at the expense of wages, reduced health care costs would mean more money left over for take-home pay. The early retiree, the widow or divorcee without a job, the employee of small business, and other people who are not members of large insured groups today would be able to buy health insurance at a reasonable cost.

CCHP would mean a loss of direct control over health benefits by labor leaders. They would no longer have this rich source of bargaining prizes. However, as we approach 100 percent employer-paid comprehensive benefits, with health costs outrunning general inflation, health benefits become an albatross around the necks of employers and union leaders, eating up an increasing percentage of total compensation and yielding no additional benefit to either. The opportunities for bargaining prizes and competitive advantages in the labor market become exhausted. By joining forces to create an effective competitive system, labor and management could get better care for workers at less cost and simplify employer-union relationships.

For the poor, CCHP offers continuity of subsidized health plan coverage that is independent of job or Medicaid eligibility. It offers access to health plans that serve the middle class and an increased supply of doctors resulting from the "capping" of demand in well-served areas. CCHP would be especially helpful to the working poor.

Medicare beneficiaries would be able to obtain protection against catastrophic medical expense and reduced or eliminated cost sharing. By joining a completely prepaid comprehensive plan, they could eliminate the unpredictability of medical costs and the complexity of claims forms they face today.

For taxpayers, CCHP offers a finite "controllable" government commitment to personal health care services versus today's open-ended commitment. It would require less of a tax increase than some of the main alternatives, less of a tax burden in the long run than would be entailed by permitting the present situation to continue developing as it has.

TWO MAJOR PROBLEMS

Government as Gatekeeper

Today, employers, unions, and trustees of labor-management health and welfare funds decide which health plans will be offered to employee groups. As noted earlier, management and labor leaders have, for the most part, sought to use their control over health benefits for their own purposes, not to create a competitive market of health plans serving the whole community. Nevertheless, there are certain advantages to having employers and unions serve as the "gatekeepers." As a part of the private sector, they can use judgments in purchasing decisions not ordinarily allowed to civil servants, who are constrained by procurement laws, and they are generally concerned with the welfare of their employees or members.

CCHP would make the government the gatekeeper, that is, the agency that would review health plans for qualification and inclusion in the enrollment process. At best, this prospect will be greeted with ambivalence by many observers. Such government control would mean susceptibility to all kinds of transient political influences, perhaps the most dangerous of which would be pressure from established health plans to keep out new competitors.

If one based one's judgment on the record of the Civil Service Commission in running the Federal Employees Health Benefits Program, one would be optimistic. For some sixteen years, the qualification process for "comprehensive plans" was managed by Marie Henderson, a tough-minded person who was not afraid to use her judgment. Thanks to her, some sixty-five plans were qualified, and they served large numbers of beneficiaries without scandal or significant financial failure. (A few small HMOs serving federal employees failed, but the program protected the employees without breaks in coverage.)

On the other hand, the HMO Act of 1973 made the Department of Health, Education, and Welfare the agency responsible for qualifying health maintenance organizations. DHEW's record has not been impressive. During 1977, the General Accounting Office evaluated fourteen of the twenty-seven HMOs that had received federal qualification by the end of 1976, finding that "3 of the 14 have a good chance of achieving financial independence within their first 5 years of operation after qualification; 5 have a fair chance; and 6 have a poor chance."[8] Since then, two of the fourteen have gone into bankruptcy. The GAO blamed "fragmented responsibility and uncoordinated efforts in operating the program, insufficient staff with expertise needed to administer the program effectively, and slow issuance of final regulations. . . ."[9] Admittedly, these were all small businesses starting up in a hostile environment, so some failures should not be surprising. But the point is that DHEW qualification does not say much about the merits of the enterprise.

In part, the difference can be explained by the fact that the Civil Service Commission had a much simpler task. It was acting as a private buyer on behalf of its beneficiaries. The ordinary procurement laws were waived. The Federal Employees' Health Benefits Program was based on the assumption that civil servants as consumers could make sensible choices for themselves. DHEW, on the other hand, was saddled with conflicting objectives and was subjected to shifting political forces. It was supposed to promote the growth of HMOs and also oversee their performance. It was supposed to carry into practical application the dreams of some health-policy thinkers who saw the HMO as "the true embodi-

ment of everything that is excellent" in health care delivery. The heavy
burdens thus placed on HMOs damaged their competitive position. Unrealistic claims for HMOs and the HMO program raised expectations that
could not be fulfilled and that led to inevitable disappointment. A vicious
cycle got going in which each HMO failure set up pressures for more
detailed regulation and paperwork—thus ensuring more failures. CCHP
could not function with a gatekeeper caught in such a political trap.

What is needed is a body that would function more like the Civil
Service Commission, perhaps an independent commission in each state
made up of representatives of employers, unions, and consumers. For
CCHP to succeed, the gatekeeper must be at least as interested in getting
good competitors into the system as in keeping bad ones out. Rather than
trying to prevent health plans from failing, the administrator of CCHP
should protect the beneficiaries from the consequences of failure of their
health plans and then let the market do its work.

Discontinuity

CCHP would keep health care delivery in the private sector, and it
would function with existing institutions operating in new ways. But in
some important respects it would represent a major change from the
present. CCHP would shift the basis for health care financing from experience-rated insurance plans serving employee groups to community-
rated financing and delivery plans open to all eligible persons in a market
area. The buyers would be consumers rather than employers. The health
plans I envision under CCHP do not exist now on a scale needed to serve
the entire population. As one friendly critic observed, "It is easier to see
how CCHP would operate, once established, than it is to see how to get
there from here." There is no reason to suppose that Blue Cross–Blue
Shield and commercial insurers would not offer qualified health plans.
But the step from here to there would be a big one. Congress usually
works in terms of "incremental changes," small steps whose short-term
implications are fairly predictable in advance. The enactment of Medicare,
Medicaid, and the Social Security Act are exceptions. This aspect of CCHP
led to requests, from members of Congress and others, for proposals for
incremental steps, possibly for trials in some areas before extending CCHP
to the whole country. This is the subject of Chapter 8.

8
Steps Toward Comprehensive Reform

The need to get the costs of health care under control is urgent. Another doubling of Medicare and Medicaid outlays will cause a severe strain on federal and state government budgets. Strong medicine is needed to correct the powerful cost-increasive forces at work today. I believe that the comprehensive Consumer Choice Health Plan proposal would be the most effective way of getting the costs under control. And I have heard no good reason for waiting.

But many people are not persuaded that we should adopt this comprehensive reform. Others may be persuaded, but believe that it cannot be enacted in one large step. But many people may be willing to try some less far-reaching steps. Members of Congress and their staffs who have studied Consumer Choice Health Plan have asked me how the principles of fair economic competition could be applied in smaller steps. This chapter outlines some of the ways.

REQUIRE EMPLOYERS TO OFFER EMPLOYEES CHOICES

The link between jobs and health insurance, fostered by the favorable tax treatment of employer-provided health benefits, has become one of the most important barriers to competition among health care financing and delivery plans. How this has happened was explained in Chapters 2 and 5. Most people are still offered a single health insurance plan by their employer and are thus denied the benefits of competition and choice. Surely Congress did not intend such a result when it enacted the Internal Revenue Code of 1954.

Congress recognized the desirability of multiple choice when it passed the Health Maintenance Organization Act of 1973, which requires employers of twenty-five or more employees to offer them the opportunity to join one group practice and one individual practice health maintenance organization if such federally qualified HMOs are available and ask to be offered. As explained in Chapter 5, this was an important step in the right direction. But it has not had a major impact on the total system. The act did not give employers any positive incentive to seek out HMOs and help them get started. Unfortunately, many employers have seen the "dual choice" requirement as an undesirable government intrusion on their prerogatives and have made it difficult for HMOs to be offered to their employees. Minimal compliance with the law can fall short of giving HMOs a truly fair chance to compete. We need stronger incentives for employers to offer their employees choices of health plan. Moreover, there are other potentially attractive health care financing and delivery systems that do not meet the detailed specifications of the HMO Act. We need a broader concept of desirable competing system.

A logical way to meet these needs would be to require every employer above a certain size to offer employees a choice of no less than three health insurance or health care delivery plans meeting minimum federal standards (see below). Different "options" from the same insurance company would not meet this requirement; real competition is the goal. The HMO Act would still apply. But if HMOs were not available, other alternative delivery systems or even traditional insurance plans would have to be offered.

A logical way to motivate employers to meet this requirement would be to make doing so a condition for continued favorable tax treatment of their health-benefits plans. That is, if an employer failed to meet this requirement after a certain date, its contributions to employee health benefits would no longer be excluded from the employees' taxable incomes. This would give employers a powerful incentive to comply; failure to do so would reduce the buying power of the dollars they spend to attract and retain employees. (The main reason for making noncomplying health benefits taxable to the employee rather than nondeductible to the employer is that many people work for employers that do not pay taxes, such as government, schools, hospitals, and other nonprofit institutions.)

I believe that a requirement of at least three choices is important to "connect the market," that is, to make it likely that the alternative delivery systems would find themselves competing with one another in a significant number of employee groups. If the requirement were simply a dual choice, it is more likely that some groups would be served by one alternative delivery system and a traditional insurance plan, while others would be served by another and traditional insurance, and the two alternative delivery systems would not meet each other in competition. This has been the case in some markets where one or two large HMOs compete with traditional insurance, but rarely with each other. Our goal should be to set off a "self-sustaining chain reaction of competition," as has occurred in Minneapolis.

There is no way of knowing whether requiring three choices will be adequate to create a truly competitive market in most communities. The result will depend in part on whether employers, once converted to the multiple-choice way of doing health insurance business, will go beyond the minimum requirements of the law where necessary to make competition effective.

If the requirement of three choices is not adequate, further measures could be taken. For example, President Carter's Phase I National Health Plan, announced in June 1979, would require all employers to offer their employees a choice among a traditional insurance plan meeting federal standards and all federally qualified HMOs in their area. Some large employers, such as Hewlett-Packard and IBM, have adopted essentially that policy on their own. Another proposal is simple "portability" of HMO membership. If an employee belongs to a federally qualified HMO and changes jobs, he or she should be allowed to keep the HMO membership and have it paid for through the new employer, even if that employer did not offer that HMO previously.

Any particular rule about a required number of choices will seem arbitrary and will not fit nicely all the many different circumstances of employers and employees. But it is important to recognize that the tax laws have put control of health benefits into the hands of employers, and for the most part this has served as a major barrier to competition. So the situation we have today is not exactly a pristine state of natural free enterprise deserving special protection. Rather, the situation we have today is the accidental by-product of tax laws that were enacted when health care costs were not the major problem they are today and the concept of competitive alternative delivery systems was practically unheard of.

Some employers complain that any requirement to offer choices of health plan would mean added complexity and extra work. Actually, the experience of those employers that have already voluntarily adopted this mode of doing business shows that very little extra work is required. They have found offering of choices to be simple and satisfactory.

The problem is not complexity; the problem is unfamiliarity. Today, employers offering employees a single insured fee-for-service plan are saying, in effect, "Go to any licensed doctor or hospital, and the cost will be paid by us." We do not hear complaints from employers about the many different doctors to whom their employees go, even though an increasing number of employers are actually processing individual claims (or paying an insurance company to do it for them).

If there were a number of competing alternative delivery systems serving the community, we would think it natural for our employers to offer us "free choice of health plan" instead of "free choice of doctor." Employers would say, in effect, "Subscribe to any licensed health plan, and the premium will be paid through payroll deduction and an employer contribution." This actually would be a much simpler way of doing business. And in such a system we would think it quite natural that when we change jobs, we would keep our membership in the health plan of our choice and merely change the source of premium contributions from the old employer to the new one. We would have moved from a system of job-centered health insurance to a system of consumer-centered health insurance. These proposals for requiring employers to offer choices would start moving us in that direction.

REQUIRE EQUAL FIXED-DOLLAR EMPLOYER CONTRIBUTIONS

The next step toward fair economic competition would be to require employer contributions to employee health insurance to be in the form of fixed dollar amounts that are the same whichever health plan the employee chooses, as explained in Chapter 5. This proposal would not require employers to contribute at any particular level; that would remain a matter for mutual agreement between employer and employees. If an employee chooses a plan that costs less than the employer's contributions, the employee should receive the difference in cash or other benefits.

There are many ways employers and unions that are not now in compliance with this principle could work out alternative arrangements that are in compliance, even without taking away already bargained benefits. One promising route would be through "cafeteria style" benefit plans. (The legal status of these plans was established by the Revenue Act of 1978.) The idea is that each employee receives a "budget" for fringe benefits, a fixed total amount. Employees who choose a less costly health plan can apply the difference to other benefits, such as retirement, or to an account for the payment of health care expenses not covered by the health plan. Such benefit plans have proved workable in practical application. (For reasons explained in Chapter 5, employees cannot be given a choice of buying no health insurance and using all of the money for other purposes.)

As noted earlier, today many of the employers that offer a choice pay 100 percent of the premium, whichever plan the employee chooses. Thus they pay more to more costly health plans and so subsidize health plans with weak cost controls against those with effective cost controls. This proposal would cause health plans to face fair economic competition. The employee who chooses a more costly health plan would have to pay the difference in cash or other benefits foregone.

STANDARDS FOR ALL HEALTH-BENEFITS PLANS

The next step toward fair economic competition would be to establish minimum standards applicable to all health plans that qualify as nontaxable fringe benefits. The first is that all health-benefits plans should be required to cover, as a minimum uniform set of benefits, the basic health services defined in the Health Maintenance Organization Act or some similar but less costly definition of comprehensive health services. The reasons for such a standard were explained in Chapter 7. The coverage could be subject to substantial copayments and deductibles, and additional benefits could be offered. This requirement would not need to increase health insurance premiums. The extra costs resulting from the addition of previously uncovered services could be offset by raising the copayments or deductibles.

The second standard that ought to be required of all tax-favored health insurance plans is a limit on direct out-of-pocket payments by the insured family, or "catastrophic-expense protection." All health plans should be required to limit consumer cost sharing for basic health services to some reasonable maximum annual amount. The reason for this is that today, tens of millions of Americans lack "catastrophic-expense protection," even though they have some health insurance. This is particularly unfortunate in view of the fact that the infrequency of catastrophic-illness expense makes this kind of insurance much less costly than "first dollar" insurance that pays a part of the first doctor bill.

The third standard is continuity of coverage. Every health-benefits plan offered by an employer ought to be required to provide continued group coverage under the plan for at least thirty days to any individual covered under the plan who would otherwise lose such coverage on account of the death, unemployment, or divorce of the employee. Such people ought to be allowed to buy continued group coverage under the plan for an additional year upon payment of premium at the group rate. No plan should be allowed to exclude or restrict coverage because of prior medical conditions. In addition, every plan should be required to offer the right to individuals who lose coverage under the group plan to convert to an individual health insurance plan covering basic health services at a reasonable premium rate.

Ideally, the standard ought to ensure the right of all those who lose their group coverage to convert to individual coverage at group-premium rates without proof of insurability or reference to prior medical conditions and to keep such coverage for as long as they need it. (This is not saying that they be given health insurance free, merely that they be allowed to continue to buy it at their own expense—a modest ideal.) The standard proposed here is much weaker than this, requiring that the continued insurance at group rates be available for only a year, because this ideal is not attainable under the present system of experience-rated insurance based on employment groups. The reasons for this were explained in Chapter 7.

Again, I believe that the best solution in the long run is to require community rating of all tax-exempt health plans. This would eliminate the difference between group and individual rates. We would not have the problem of people being unable to buy health insurance at reasonable premium rates if most of the people in each community were served by several alternative delivery systems, each of which practiced community rating—which means spreading the medical risks over the whole enrolled population. Then, in effect, each health care plan would carry its own former group members. Indeed, at least some of the large prototype HMOs do offer former group members the right to buy an individual conversion policy at the community rate and to continue membership as long as they want it.

FREEDOM OF CHOICE IN MEDICARE

The Medicare reforms described in Chapter 7 could be enacted without enactment of the rest of Consumer Choice Health Plan. Indeed, there have been proposals to do just this (see below). The first step, which has been proposed by the Carter administration, would be to permit Medicare beneficiaries to designate that an amount equal to their adjusted average per capita cost (or 95 percent of it) be paid to the health maintenance organization of their choice as a fixed premium contribution. Alternatively, this same option could be allowed for a broader class of private health plans. A more far-reaching possibility would be simply to replace Medicare, for new beneficiaries becoming eligible as of a certain date with a whole new system modeled after the Federal Employees Health Benefits Program.

A LIMIT ON TAX-FREE EMPLOYER CONTRIBUTIONS

Another possible incremental step would be to put a limit on the amount of employer contribution to health benefits that could be tax free to the employee. In other words, Congress might continue to exempt from taxes an amount of employer contribution sufficient to pay for a comprehensive health care plan of good quality, economically provided, but require that above that amount, people pay the extra cost of more costly health plans out of their own net after-tax incomes.

This would correct the cost-increasing incentives in the tax laws described in Chapter 2. It would mean that above the limit, people would be paying for health benefits with after-tax rather than before-tax dollars, so they would be motivated to demand more value for each extra dollar of premium payment.

In the absence of the comprehensive reforms described in Chapter 7, such a limit would raise at least two problems. The first is that there are wide regional differences in health care costs, as described in Chapter 7. In principle, there could be different limits in different states, reflecting the different costs, along the lines described in Chapter 7. Although this would be somewhat more complex than a flat across-the-board limit, it would not be more complex than many other provisions of the tax laws.

The second problem stems from the widespread use of experience rating of health insurance premiums. This means that some groups may be receiving larger employer contributions not because they have more generous health benefits or have chosen a more costly style of care, but simply because they are less healthy as a group, possibly because of age or occupation. A small group might be hard-hit by one or a few catastrophic-illness cases. Such people would have a legitimate argument that their limit on tax-free employer contributions ought to reflect their greater than average medical need.

I believe that the only practical answer to this problem in the long run is to require that all tax-subsidized health plans practice community rating, thereby spreading medical risks over all of the insured groups. Thus the limit on tax-free employer contributions may have to await the requirement of community rating.

FAVORABLE RESPONSE FROM KEY MEMBERS OF CONGRESS

The principles underlying these proposals have received a favorable response from several members of the congressional committees having jurisdiction over health care financing policy. These people have applied the principles of fair economic competition in the development of their own proposals.

In June 1979 Representative Al Ullman, Chairman of the Ways and Means Committee, told a Washington conference on health policy: "Government simply cannot regulate the entire industry effectively. Once the accelerator is stuck, putting on the brakes may slow the car—but the damage is extensive. We can, however, identify the cost to the consumer and foster keener competition."[1] Then he outlined a proposal to:

reverse the incentives created by our tax system to select the most expensive health care coverage. . . . create incentives for employees and employers to choose plans that contain cost incentive features. . . . encourage, and ultimately force, employers to offer their employees a choice between plans that are prepaid and plans with substantial copayment features. . . . change the incentives in medicare to encourage elderly patients to select prepaid plans rather than the fee-for-service system.[2]

In October Mr. Ullman introduced the Health Cost Restraint Act of 1979.[3]

In July Senator David Durenberger, a member of the Health Subcommittee of the Finance Committee, introduced the Health Incentives Reform Act of 1979 (HIRA). In the accompanying statement, he said:

> I am proposing a program which rewards providers for delivering better care at less cost and which rewards consumers for choosing better quality care at lower premiums. The basic principle of HIRA is that the option to choose among competing health care alternatives can lower prices and improve medical care coverage. Competitive incentives, which operate effectively in other sectors of the economy, can work in health care if we plan with reasonable forethought.[4]

One important thing Representative Ullman and Senator Durenberger have in common is that they have both observed effective health-plan competition in their home districts. Ullman's district includes Clackamas County, Oregon, where the Physicians Association of Clackamas County competes with the Kaiser-Permanente Medical Care Program. In Senator Durenberger's home state of Minnesota, seven health maintenance organizations compete and serve more than 300,000 people in the Twin Cities, as we saw in Chapter 5. Both men have studied these situations carefully and have seen in them lessons that could be applied to the whole country.

Also in June Senator Richard Schweiker, ranking minority member of the Health and Scientific Research Subcommittee of the Labor and Human Resources Committee, announced a comprehensive health-reform plan. He said:

> Our health insurance system now resembles a free lunch arrangement for doctors and hospitals. They order the tests and provide the equipment. Then the insurance companies pay the bills and later pass the cost on to consumers in the form of higher insurance premiums. . . . We can take action to break this inflationary spiral by giving health care consumers incentives, in the form of health insurance premium rebates, so they become more active in health care pricing decisions, and by ensuring that they have competitive health insurance alternatives to choose from. . . . My plan will give consumers new opportunities and new rewards for taking action themselves, through the private marketplace, against health cost inflation.[5]

And also in June 1979, Representative David Stockman, a member of the Health and Environment Subcommittee of the Interstate and Foreign Commerce Committee, wrote:

> What is required is merely the conversion of open-ended service coverage entitlements into fixed monetary contributions by either government or em-

ployer payors to one of a multiple choice of plans available to each consumer. . . . the activation of 150 million adult health care shoppers would dramatically transform the medical marketplace. In order to market their services efficiently, health care providers would find it necessary to organize themselves into total service delivery agencies. . . ."[6]

Bills have been introduced to implement these ideas. The incentives-and-competition approach to cost control has been established as a serious contender to become the basis for health care financing policy.

FURTHER STEPS

Taken together, incremental steps such as these could take us a long way toward a system of universal coverage by competing private health care plans with built-in incentives for consumer satisfaction and cost control. Problems would remain, but they could be handled by subsequent legislation.

As we have seen, our ability to achieve cost control through economic competition, as well as our ability to achieve universal coverage at affordable costs, are blocked by today's widespread practices of experience rating and preferred-risk selection. As long as these practices are allowed, some health plans will seek to compete by limiting their coverage to preferred-risk groups to whom they can charge a lower premium, instead of competing by organizing and delivering services more economically. Preferred-risk selection is a way to escape from competitive pressure to control cost.

The opposite of experience rating and preferred-risk selection is community rating and open enrollment. Community rating by itself does not solve much if health plans can systematically restrict their membership to healthy people. The Health Maintenance Organization Act of 1973 attempted to impose open enrollment and community rating on health maintenance organizations, which served less than 3 percent of the population, while leaving untouched the systems serving the other 97 percent. If these requirements had been applied, they would have killed HMOs by requiring them to accept the high-risk people who could not get coverage from the rest of the system. The leading HMOs chose not to participate in the program until the law was amended, in 1976, to limit sharply the open-enrollment requirement and to allow newly qualified HMOs to experience rate.

If we want to cure the problems arising from experience rating and preferred-risk selection, we should seek to move the entire system toward one in which community rating and open enrollment are uniformly applied to all health plans. One way this could be done is through phased tax incentives. Over a period of years, the government might gradually reduce the percentage of employer premium contributions that are tax-free for health plans that do not community rate and that do not engage in specified open-enrollment practices.

When the majority of people are served by community-rated comprehensive-care organizations, the step to a universal system such as Consumer Choice Health Plan will appear much smaller than it appears today.

The incremental steps discussed so far are all proposals for action by the federal government. It is logical to focus on the federal government because the main perverse incentives arise from federal laws. Moreover, the federal government is the agency most likely to be motivated to act to change the system because rising health care costs are having such a large effect on the federal budget. However, there are many very constructive actions that could be taken by state, and even local, governments and by private-sector employers.

California has a multiple-choice health plan system for its employees, similar to the Federal Employees Program. The statute has a provision allowing local government agencies to join that system. So far, the incentives to join have not been very strong, and relatively few have done so. The state government could greatly enhance health plan competition if it were to strengthen the incentives for local government agencies to join the state's system and, at the same time, to seek out and include new competing health plans so that there would be several alternative delivery systems in each service area. The cost to a new alternative delivery system to get started would be greatly reduced if, by satisfying the requirements of one managing agency, it could have access to such a large market as all public-sector employees in its service area. Other states could proceed along the same lines.

Local government agencies could join together and create the same kind of multiple-choice system. To do so would not only save them considerable administrative costs, but also, again, reduce the start-up costs for new health care plans.

Private employers in each of many market areas could emulate the enlightened actions of leading Minneapolis employers such as General Mills, Control Data, Honeywell, and Cargill. These companies studied the problem of health care costs together, decided to offer fair multiple choice, and agreed to help new alternative delivery systems to get started. Employers in many other areas could decide to do the same thing.

CONCLUDING REMARKS

"Is the fulfillment of these ideas a visionary hope? Have they insufficient roots in the motives which govern the evolution of political society?" John Maynard Keynes asked these questions in 1935 about his most influential book.[7] And I do wonder whether it is possible to achieve an "industrial revolution" in health care services in the United States in the 1980s.

The interests arrayed against it are formidable. Control over health benefits has given labor leaders an apparently inexhaustible source of bargaining prizes with persuasive emotional appeal. It has given employers an instrument with which to compete more effectively in the labor market and to bind employees more closely to their firms. The private health insurance industry is presently based on concepts antithetical to those I am recommending: cost reimbursement rather than cost control and financial intermediation rather than organization, management, and delivery of health care services. The medical profession has profited greatly, in money and in freedom, from insured fee for service. The hospital industry has grown comfortable and secure in cost reimbursement. And many of the "Washington health policy establishment" find their whole *raison d'être* in an ever more pervasive system of regulation.

Still, there are powerful forces making for change. The growth in costs of health services will force the government to act. The almost unbroken record of failure of regulation of health care on the public-utility model and public disenchantment with expanding bureaucracy make it unattractive to pursue that course.

Moreover, various interested parties are finding that a continuation of present trends will not be to their advantage. As health benefits have become more comprehensive in more companies, they have become a less effective tool for management to use in competing for employees. And new opportunities for bargaining prizes for union leaders are becoming exhausted. The rapidly increasing cost of health benefits uses money that could otherwise go to the workers in wages.

More and more employers are discovering how little their third-party insurer is really contributing to cost control, and they are switching to self-insured plans, sometimes contracting with the insurance carrier to provide claims-processing services. So the health insurance business is slipping away from the insurance companies. Some of the leading companies, such as Prudential, Connecticut General, INA, and SAFECO, are actively developing alternative delivery systems to position themselves for a market of health plan competition. Nationally, Blue Cross–Blue Shield is involved in some sixty-six alternative delivery system developments.

Some physicians recognize that the status quo is untenable, and they would greatly prefer economic competition in the private sector to increased regulation. The leaders of the hospital associations, both voluntary and investor-owned, have looked at the public-utility regulation future and found it wanting. Given the choice between regulation and competition, for the most part they are supporting the latter.

But the most formidable barriers to "the fulfillment of these ideas" are not vested interests; they are the ideas that now shape the thinking of most people. The casualty-insurance model of health care financing is deeply entrenched in the public mind, not only in this country but in Canada and Europe as well. Health maintenance organizations receive attention from time to time, either in a wave of congressional enthusiasm about cost control or as some television reporter seeks to portray the unusual for the audience. But the idea soon fades from the national consciousness, perceived as a unique phenomenon, applicable only in special places such as the West Coast and Minnesota. The link between jobs and health insurance is another unquestioned fixed point in most people's thinking. It is difficult for them to conceive of a system of multiple choice of health plans, because it is outside of their experience. And the public-utility model seems natural to this "charitable" industry. How else to explain the renewal of costly laws such as the Health Planning Act and programs such as PSROs after such evidence of their failure?

At this point, I think that the best hope lies with employers and in the leadership of people such as Congressman Ullman and Senator Durenberger, who have seen health plan competition work in their districts and who believe that it could be made to work on a national scale. If the employers in any of a dozen or more communities where strong alternative delivery systems already exist were to apply systematically the principles of fair multiple choice, they could create the kind of health plan competition we have seen in Minneapolis and Hawaii. More members of Congress would be impressed by the favorable development in their home districts.

Keynes also concluded, "But, soon or late, it is ideas, not vested interests, which are dangerous for good or evil."[8] And surely there is nothing like experience to sell an idea.

APPENDIX
SUMMARY AND ANALYSIS
OF OTHER LEADING
NATIONAL HEALTH
INSURANCE PROPOSALS

There have been many national health insurance proposals over the past decade. Eighteen bills were introduced in the 94th Congress (1975-1976) alone.[1] The proposals can be grouped into a few broad categories, each with many variations, some of which are nonessential from the point of view of this book. It is essential to any national health insurance plan that there be one legally established definition of covered basic health services that serves as a minimum standard for all participating health care plans. Whether or not a particular service is included in the list may not be essential. Generally speaking, any of a number of definitions could be incorporated into any of the bills. (From the point of view of the providers of some services, however, whether those services are in or out may be the most important issue.) The proposals keep changing in detail, so that an exposition of many of the details would be confusing.

What would seem useful to the general reader is a summary description and analysis of three basic models, broad concepts of organization and finance into which the main alternatives other than CCHP fit. These may be characterized as: (1) the Kennedy plans; (2) mandated employer-provided insurance for the employed and public insurance for all others; and (3) government as universal third-party payor.

There is an important fourth alternative, "catastrophic health insurance" as proposed by Senators Russell Long and Abraham Ribicoff. The "Long-Ribicoff" proposal has quite limited objectives; it does not address the overall structure of the health care financing and delivery system or the problem of control of cost, which is the subject of this book. If it were enacted, the overall structure of the industry would resemble today's or the "employer-provided insurance" model described below.

The dividing lines among these approaches are not precise. To some extent, they merge into one another, or one would be likely to evolve into another. Elements of one can be included in another, and an unlimited number of new plans can thereby be generated.

THE KENNEDY PLANS

Although Senator Edward M. Kennedy's statements emphasize making comprehensive health care services available to all Americans, without regard to ability to pay, and distributing the cost of health care equitably, these goals could be achieved in the context of several broad frameworks for financing and organization. What really distinguishes the Kennedy plans from the others is their emphasis on fundamental reform of the financing and delivery system through comprehensive government controls. These comprehensive health insurance plans would shift health care finance from the fee-for-service, cost-reimbursement, casualty-insurance model to a system in which all health care providers would work within a budget set in advance by government.

The first Kennedy plan, called the Health Security Act, was introduced in 1970.[2] In 1974 Senator Kennedy joined with Congressman Wilbur Mills to introduce the Comprehensive National Health Insurance Act of 1974. "Kennedy-Mills," as it was known, was based on the model of government as universal third-party payor (see below).[3] It was a temporary effort by Senator Kennedy to find an acceptable compromise with people who wanted national health insurance, but were unwilling to accept the far-reaching controls of Health Security. In April 1978 Kennedy announced that he and the labor leaders associated with him were preparing a major new plan, the full details of which were published in May 1979.[4] To understand the new proposal, one must begin with the first one.

Health Security

Health Security was designed to change health care financing from today's open-ended payment of provider bills after the fact to a system in which all providers would have to live within budgets set in advance, within a total determined by Congress. The act would have assigned the entire financing and management of health insurance to the federal government. The act levied taxes on payrolls, self-employed and unearned income, and required matching this with an equal sum from federal general revenues. A federal Health Security Board would have established an annual national budget, based on the cost of the program in the preceding year, adjusted for changes in prices, population, and number of providers. The budget could not exceed total projected receipts. Thus there would be a firm lid on total health care spending.

The Board would allocate the budget to each region, based on the previous year's allocation, modified for prices, population, and number of providers. At the regional level, the allocations would be divided into categories for institutional services, physicians' services, dental services, drugs, appliances, and other services. The regional funds would be allocated on a similar basis to health-service areas. The Board would be directed to reduce gradually, and ultimately to eliminate, differences among the regions in real per capita spending on health services.

Within these budgeted totals, the Board would then contract for covered services with participating providers who agreed to make no charge directly to the patient for covered services. General hospitals, skilled-nursing homes, home-health agencies, and other institutional providers would be paid on the basis of annual budgets negotiated with the Board. HMOs would receive a per capita amount established for the geographic area for the range of covered services offered, for persons enrolled with them. Physicians and other professionals could be paid by fee-for-service, capitation, or salary. Fee schedules would be negotiated with medical societies. The funds budgeted for physicians and other professionals would be allocated to those selecting salary, capitation, and fee for service. If, during the year, total payments for fee for service were greater than allocated, the amount of fees would be reduced proportionately, much as occurs in an individual practice association.

New facilities could not be built unless approved by state health-planning agencies or the Board.

The bill directed the Department of Health, Education, and Welfare and the Board to do planning to improve the supply and distribution of personnel and facilities and the organization of health services. Recent versions of Health Security adopted health planning as prescribed in the National Health Planning and Resources Development Act of 1974. Priority financial assistance would be given to improving outpatient services when provided as part of a coordinated system of comprehensive care, including group practice organizations and public or nonprofit comprehensive-care centers.

In brief, Health Security would have created a centrally and politically controlled system in which all participating providers would get all of their money from tax revenues through the federal government. Spending for personal health care services would be set in the political process on the basis of national priorities rather than in the marketplace based on individual priorities.

Health Security had important strengths. Its authors recognized, correctly in my view, that costs could not be controlled without a fundamental and comprehensive reform of the delivery system. Piecemeal controls are bound to fail. It sought to reorganize health services into comprehensive-care systems. It sought equity in the use of public funds, and it sought to equalize per capita spending among regions and between HMOs and the fee-for-service sector.

The main failing of Health Security was that in the real world of our democratic political system, it could not have achieved its goals. The government cannot reorganize the health care system by direct controls. Providers and consumers would resist changes that they did not perceive to be in their interest. Experience with other regulated industries, and with national health insurance in other countries, suggests that total government control would fix the system in the patterns that exist now. The full political and financial power of the established health care and related interests would be arrayed against change. For example, it has been extremely difficult for government to close unneeded Public Health Service hospitals, defense installations, and schools. Government attempts to close hospitals in overbedded areas would drown in a deluge of political pressure and lawsuits from employee and citizen groups. Imagine the vested interests and rigidity surrounding the allocations among hospitals, doctors, dentists, and other providers. The Health Security Act seemed almost designed to freeze existing allocations and to protect existing jobs.

The Health Security Act proposed to bring total spending under control by "top-down budgeting." Top-down budgeting may indeed bring total spending under control. But of itself (without something like the incentives provided by competition), the mechanism has no built-in means for ensuring that providers of services put much creativity, or even cooperation, into living within the budget and doing the best possible job for consumers.

This pessimistic assessment is borne out by the experience in our largest public health care systems. A recent National Academy of Sciences study of the Veterans Administration (VA) Health Care System concluded:

> The data show that the geographic distribution of hospital beds is not in accord with the geographic variation in demand for hospital care. The data also suggest that there are too many acute beds being operated in the system . . . about half the patients in acute medical beds, one-third of the patients in surgical beds, and well over half the patients in psychiatric beds do not require—and are not receiving—the acute care services associated with these types of beds. These data provide additional evidence that many more VA hospital beds are being operated than are required to meet the needs of veterans. . . . The VA has installed many expensive specialized medical facilities that, in many hospitals, are used at rates far below their capacity. Furthermore, in many communities in which VA hospitals have underutilized services, there are community hospitals offering the same services, and the community facilities are frequently being utilized at rates well below their capacity.[5]

A recent study of the military health care system showed that the Defense Department operates and fills far too many beds. As the report tactfully phrased it, "the incentives in workload-based programming may encourage relatively heavy use of inpatient care."[6] The point is that in the bureaucratic budgeting system, one strengthens one's case for more by doing a poor job with the budget one has. Providers can "prove" that they need larger budgets by pointing to waiting lines and other evidence of poor service.

The government is simply incapable of managing the whole health care system very well. There is no precedent to suggest that it can. The great government managerial successes such as the space program were "heroic" crash efforts, done in an atmosphere of great urgency in which the usual rules were suspended. The government does not have the necessary management personnel and organization to run the health care system, and there is good reason to believe that it could not acquire them on a sustained basis. The Health Security Board might attract outstanding management talent to begin with, based on dedication to public service. But when it became clear that doing an effective job means doing things like closing excess acute hospitals in some areas to pay for needed facilities in others, and Board members started feeling the wrath of citizens expressed through their Congressmen and seeing the implementation of their plans tied up in court, the two-year turnover typical of Assistant Secretaries in the Defense Department and the Department of Health, Education, and Welfare would be sure to emerge.

Many things about government make for high turnover among top executives, including the unfortunate politics of executive pay, which squeeze out people with attractive private-sector alternatives, and the political-reward system, which is more sensitive to appearances than to day-to-day performance. Public-sector managers are subject to many complex procedural rules and to being overruled by political leaders for short-term political purposes. Running a large organization effectively requires long-term commitment by its managers; it cannot be done well on revolving two- to four-year tours.

Health Security was abandoned in the spring of 1978 because its authors recognized that it did not fit with some of the basic political requirements of the times. These included the need to hold down the costs appearing on the federal budget, the need to allow private insurers to retain a major role in health care, and the need to limit the size and scope of government activity.

Health Care for All Americans

The new Kennedy plan, Health Care for All Americans, announced in May 1979, is not easy to summarize concisely. It appears to be a complex mix of: "top-down budgeting" by government agencies at the federal and state levels, similar to Health Security; collective bargaining among providers, insurers, and purchasers of health insurance (employers, unions, and representatives of individual consumers); regulation of providers on the public-utility model by both the federal and state governments; and competition in the private sector.

At the top would be the National Health Board, an independent federal agency reporting to the President. It would establish national policy and oversee implementation. It would organize and supervise the processes of budget preparation and negotiations over payments to providers and insurers at the national and state levels. It would certify participating insurers. And it would contract with State Health Boards.

The State Health Boards would be public corporations, with members appointed by the governors, that would prepare and submit annual state health budgets to the National Board and implement the budgets as approved. These budgets would provide payment for all of the services within each state covered by the law. State Boards would organize and supervise a negotiating process among providers, insurers, and purchasers of health insurance, governing budgets for hospitals and other institutional providers and fee schedules for doctors. The State Board would have the final authority for approval of provider budgets.

There would be four kinds of insurers: commercial insurance companies, Blue Cross–Blue Shield, individual practice HMOs, and prepaid group practice HMOs. To participate, each insurer would have to agree to assume responsibility for paying for at least the comprehensive benefits specified in the law for a negotiated per capita amount called a "community-rated premium." Participating insurers would also have to agree to an annual open enrollment at which they would accept all eligible persons who wanted to enroll. There would be no copayments or deductibles. Insurers would pay providers at or below the rates negotiated by providers, insurers, and purchasers. Insurers would be allowed to offer "limited provider plans," under which beneficiaries would agree to get their comprehensive benefits from selected providers offering reduced prices or other special arrangements.

Insurers would establish and join one of four consortia, national organizations with state branches, one for each type of insurer. These national corporations would act as financial clearing houses, receiving revenues and disbursing funds to member carriers and HMOs according to formulas reflecting the predicted medical needs of the population covered by each insurer. They would represent their members at the national and state-level negotiations.

Participating providers would have to agree to accept negotiated fees and budgets as payment in full. Providers would send elected representatives to national and state-level negotiations. They would be "at risk"; that is to say, if insurers in a state found that they were exceeding their budgeted totals for physician services, the State Board could require the physicians to accept a pro rata reduction in fees.

Employers would offer their employees a choice of at least one insurance plan and one HMO, and they would facilitate annual enrollment for employees and dependents. They would pay, either alone or jointly with employees, amounts called "wage-related premium payments." These payments would be required by law and would be equal to a fixed percentage of payrolls. The funds would be paid to insurers through the consortia. The authors of the plan do not consider these required payments to be taxes, because they are paid to the consortia, which are private organizations. The plan is designed this way to avoid the need for additional taxes and to keep the spending off the federal budget. This device will raise some fine legal questions about control of and accountability for the funds. Many people will find it difficult to resist referring to the required payments as "payroll taxes," and economists will consider them equivalent to payroll taxes from the point of view of economic impact.

Employed people would enroll in the health insurance plan of their choice from those offered by the employer. They would pay a part of the "wage-related premium" unless the employer agreed to pay it all. Individuals not employed and not poor would enroll in the health insurance plan of their choice. (Apparently they would be allowed a choice of any certified plan in their area, whereas employees could be limited to a choice of two.) They would pay an "income-related premium payment" integrated with their estimated personal income tax payments. These payments would not exceed the "community-rated premium" for families of the same size.

Various existing public utility-type controls would remain in operation and even be extended. State governments would prepare and propose to the State Health Boards Five-Year Plans for Health Resources Distribution. And they would implement certificate-of-need programs. Professional Standards Review Organizations would review all utilization under the program.

The main sources of funds would be the following: (1) "wage-related premiums," a flat percentage of total payrolls, calculated by the National Board and paid by employers, with possible sharing by employees; (2) "income-related premiums," paid by people with more than $2000 per person in nonwage income and set at one-half the percentage levied on payrolls; (3) per capita payments by the federal government on behalf of Supplemental Security Income recipients and by the state governments on behalf of welfare recipients; (4) Medicare payroll taxes and premiums; and (5) federal general revenues. The federal government would guarantee the consortia that they would receive their "negotiated community rates" multiplied by the applicable number of people, even if the other revenue sources were not adequate.

The process would work roughly as follows. Each State Board would prepare an annual budget for all covered services in its state. It would start with existing patterns of expenditures and would adjust them for population changes, inflation, desired changes prescribed by the state's Five-Year Health Resources Distribution plan, and other factors. The Board would submit this budget to the National Health Board.

The National Health Board would review state budgets for conformity with national guidelines. For example, the annual increase in the total of all state budgets would not be allowed to exceed the average percentage growth in the gross national product over the prior three years. In a state where per capita spending was above the national average, the rate of increase in spending would have to be below the national average. In a state where per capita spending was below the national average, spending would be allowed to increase faster. In this way per capita spending would gradually be equalized among the different regions. If Congress passed a law mandating new benefits, the National Board would build the cost into the state budgets. If proposed state budgets exceeded the limit, reductions would be directed.

The National Health Board would then calculate the percentages of payroll and nonwage income that would be needed to pay for the budgeted amounts, along with other sources of revenue. This would become the national "tax rate" for the coming year.

With its budget approved, the State Health Board would convoke a "State Negotiating Group" of providers, insurers, and purchasers of insurance to negotiate hospital budgets and physician fees. If they agreed on budgets and fees that produced a total estimated expenditure less than the approved state budget, the payroll and income-related premium rates would be reduced proportionately below the national percentages. This is to motivate the payors in each state to bargain hard.

The National Health Boards would negotiate with the consortia to establish "negotiated community-rated premiums" for each state or area. The consortia would act as clearing houses, collecting the premiums from employers, receiving payments from the federal and state governments, and paying their members the "negotiated community-rated premiums" times the number of enrollees. (The premiums would be actuarially adjusted by the consortia for the age and sex composition of the population served by each plan and any other factors considered important to predicting medical need.) If an insurer could provide or pay for the covered services for less than the "negotiated community-rated premiums," it could use the excess for any combination of retained earnings, more benefits, or tax-free cash rebates to enrollees (or, in some cases, to employers). If the insurer's costs exceeded the per capita payments, the insurer would have to absorb the loss.

The new Kennedy plan includes some elements of competition in the private sector. People are offered choices, although employed people may be offered a choice limited to one insurer and one HMO. Those who choose less costly plans get to keep the savings, in the form of either additional health benefits or cash rebates. (This is an important change from Health Security.) All competitors are subject to the same rules. Alternative delivery systems and "limited provider plans" offered by insurers are allowed to compete. Indeed, some have described the new plan as an attempt to reconcile Health Security with the principles of Consumer Choice Health Plan.

But in fact, in this plan the scope of competition would be very limited. The competitors would be constrained by many controls of various types. All of the ceilings, negotiated provider budgets and fees, and public utility–type controls make it clear that the authors of the plan place little or no confidence in the way the private sector allocates resources. All capital investment funds would be allocated by the State Boards. Hospitals would not even be allowed to receive the cash flow from depreciation allowances.

Such political control of capital would act as a major barrier to the startup and expansion of new competitors. Suppose that a group of physicians wanted to start a new prepaid group practice, housed in a new medical center, in an area already adequately supplied with facilities. Suppose that their intent was to take business away from less efficient, less attractive providers. How would they get permission from the State Health Board? They would be told that their services and facilities were not "needed." (Recall the response of the health-planning authorities to Kaiser's application to start its own heart surgery unit, described in Chapter 6.) How would they get the capital? The capital budget for each area would doubtless be allocated in "fair shares" according to existing patterns. This is typical of such politically controlled systems. The established provider interests can see to that. They have both the votes and the money. The would-be new competitor would have no members, no employees, and probably insufficient funds with which to overcome the political influence of the established providers. So the new competitor would be denied access to capital.

For a true competitive market to exist, it must be feasible, economically and politically, for new competitors to enter the market and for some existing competitors to expand at the expense of others. In the private-market system, a new competitor can risk its own capital, invest in facilities, and start selling services to customers without a certification by government that the services are "needed." Existing providers whose business is threatened by the new competitor do not have the political tools to block the new entrant. In contrast to this, the new Kennedy plan is a description of the kind of tightly controlled situation in which real innovation and delivery system reform would be impossible.

How would such a system actually work in practice? What would it look like? It is difficult to judge something so complex in concept, with so many overlapping and interrelated parts. For one thing, there are no practical examples in actual operation on which to base such a judgment. It does not appear that anything quite like it exists. The uncertainty is increased by the fact that a great deal of the workings of the system are left to regulations to be developed by the National Health Board.

One thing we can be sure of is that it would not be run as a model of rational analytical management. The management tools do not exist. Nobody knows how to set hospital budgets by analytical criteria related to the needs of the people to be cared for. Such criteria have not been developed by the National Health Service in Britain or by the Defense Department or the Veterans Administration in this country. Cost-effectiveness analysis in medical care is in a very early stage of development. HMOs with hospitals allocate hospital resources by judgment based on experience, not by the sorts of formulas that would stand up as "objective" in a political process. The only known government method, and the one that would surely be applied, is to grant each hospital for next year's budget an amount equal to this year's budget adjusted for inflation and some average population and technology growth factors.

Consider the following illustrative situation. Suppose that the average allowable increase in hospital spending in some year is 10 percent. One hospital wants a 20 percent increase and marshals all of its evidence to support it. It can only get the 20 percent increase if other hospitals are held to less than 10 percent. So the other hospitals are under pressure to prove that they need more. The number of possible ways they might go about doing this is very large. There is no objective formula for deciding such a matter. There is no consensus of experts on the correct way to reach such a decision, and there is not likely to be one soon. So the matter must be a negotiated compromise. And the likely outcome is agreement on a 10 percent increase for each hospital. In fact, the proposal is filled with devices for extrapolating from today's patterns, with changes for population and inflation. One good predictor of the health care system ten years later would be today's system, with all spending increased in proportion to the gross national product.

Finally, the bureaucratic politics of the budgetary process would doubtless play an important part in the life of the program. As noted earlier, in this kind of system providers can make the case that they need more resources by doing a poor job with what they have. They can keep people in the hospital longer and point to high occupancy as a reason for a greater budget, as happens in the Defense Department and the Veterans Administration. They can keep people waiting to generate political pressure for more resources. What is lacking in such a system are positive incentives for providers to do a better job at lower cost.

The state and national negotiations with providers over fees and budgets would have the effect of uniting the providers in their own interest. The physicians would be under strong pressure to form a powerful and tight organization for bargaining purposes. This result would be completely antithetical to the notion of the physicians' participating in competing economic units.

As to costs, the estimates prepared for the new Kennedy plan indicate, for fiscal year 1983, in 1980 dollars, total spending for services covered by the plan of $171 billion under present law, $211 billion under the Kennedy plan, for an increase of $40 billion. In terms of "on budget" federal cost, present law would provide for $51 billion for services covered by the plan, whereas the Kennedy plan would cost $80 billion, for a difference of $29 billion. Whether or not one considers that to be the true increase in the "federal budget" depends on sophisticated judgments about the difference between a tax and a compulsory "wage-related premium" that has many of the attributes of a tax, and the difference between a direct federal expenditure of such funds, and one that is indirect, but mandated by the government and under federal control.

MANDATED EMPLOYER-PROVIDED INSURANCE FOR THE EMPLOYED AND PUBLIC INSURANCE FOR ALL OTHERS

The second national health insurance model is mandated employer-provided insurance for people with jobs and public insurance for everyone else. This was the model for the Comprehensive Health Insurance Act of 1974 proposed by President Nixon and also the model for President Carter's Phase I National Health Plan proposal of 1979.

The Nixon Proposal[7]

The Nixon proposal would have established a three-part national program including: (1) an employee health-benefits plan meeting certain standards; (2) a state-operated "assisted" health care program providing coverage for low-income families and for high-risk families and employment groups; and (3) a federal health care program for the aged—in effect, expanded Medicare.

The employee plan would require employers to offer full-time employees a standardized health-benefits plan including hospital, medical, and preventive services and protection against catastrophic illness. Coverage would be implemented through private health insurance and financed through employer and employee premium contributions, with temporary federal subsidies for firms with unusually high increases in premium costs resulting from the law. Employers would be required to contribute 75 percent of the premiums. Coverage would continue, with full employer contribution, for at least ninety days after an employee's termination of work. The employee could continue it another ninety days at his or her own expense. Exclusions for preexisting conditions and waiting periods would not be allowed. Cost sharing would be related to income on a sliding scale and for the highest income group would be limited to a $150 annual deductible per person, 25 percent coinsurance, with an individual annual maximum of $1050, and a family maximum of $1500.

The state-operated assisted plan was designed to make health insurance available to all persons not otherwise insured. All persons would be eligible except those eligible for employer coverage and having incomes over specified levels and the aged. There would be income-related deductibles, coinsurance, and a maximum limit on each family's annual liability. Premiums would be income-related and tied to the state average for the employee plan. The assisted plan would be subsidized by the state and federal governments on a sliding scale, averaging 75 percent federal.

Medicare coverage would be broadened, and cost sharing would be income-related, with a maximum individual liability of $750 per year.

All enrollees would be issued health cards, and an account would be established for each enrollee. Full participating providers, those accepting payment at state-regulated rates, would be reimbursed in full by the health plan, which would then bill the beneficiary for the cost sharing. Other providers could charge more, but would have to collect from the patient the difference between the carrier's share of the regulated fee and their charge. Credit would be extended to patients at regulated interest rates to help them pay their direct costs.

As well as offering an insurance plan meeting the standards, employers would be required to offer their employees a prepaid group practice plan and an individual practice association plan, unless none was available in the area. The employer would have to offer to make a premium contribution to each of these plans at least equal to that required under the insurance. The "assisted" program and the Medicare program also would have an "HMO option," whereby the average cost to the public program could be paid to the HMO of the beneficiary's choice, with the beneficiary paying the rest of the premium.

The Carter Proposal[8]

The Carter proposal would have: (1) created a unified federal program, called HealthCare, to serve the aged and disabled, low-income people, and others who could not obtain private coverage; and (2) required employers to offer employees private health insurance meeting federal standards.

Under "the employer guarantee," all employers would have to provide full-time workers and their families with a health insurance plan covering a comprehensive list of services similar to those covered by Medicare. Large deductibles and copayments would be allowed, to help keep premium costs down, but no individual or family would face cost sharing (direct payments of its own) in excess of $2500 per year for covered services. Thus every family of an employed worker would have full protection against catastrophic medical expense. Coinsurance and deductibles would not be allowed in the case of prenatal care, delivery, and infant care.

Coverage would be implemented through private health insurance and financed through employer and employee premium contributions. Employers would be required to pay at least 75 percent of the premium cost for a plan meeting the minimum federal standards. But employers would not be required to spend more than 5 percent of payroll on such insurance. Employers facing higher costs could either buy the coverage from HealthCare at subsidized rates or obtain premium subsidies for private insurance from HealthCare. There would also be subsidies to help low-income families pay their share. There would be no waiting period for coverage after the tenth week of employment, and coverage would have to continue at least ninety days after the employee's termination of employment. After that, employees and/or dependents would have the right to buy comparable individual coverage from the insurance carrier or, if that were not available, from HealthCare.

HealthCare would replace Medicare and Medicaid and would cover a comprehensive list of services. In the case of the aged and disabled, cost sharing would be limited to $1250 per person per year. If their income, net of medical expenses, was below 55 percent of the poverty line, they would face no cost sharing. Other low-income people would become eligible for HealthCare coverage, with no cost sharing, either through becoming eligible for cash assistance or because their income, net of medical expenses, fell below 55 percent of the poverty line.

Physicians serving HealthCare beneficiaries would have to agree to accept HealthCare fees as full payment. Initially, the fee schedule would be based on Medicare averages; subsequently, it would be negotiated with physician representatives.

This approach to universal health insurance has some important strengths that have made it appealing to two presidents. It fits in with the accepted casualty insurance and public-utility models of health care financing and cost control. It does not require selling any radical new ideas. It makes maximum use of existing capabilities and existing relationships between employers and insurance companies. It is the most conservative approach, the one with the greatest continuity with present ways of doing business, likely to encounter the least opposition from established interest groups. It keeps most management and underwriting in the private sector.

Its cost to the federal budget can be low, which gives it political appeal. It avoids the need for a large tax increase or for required payments that look like taxes. (Although a "mandated employer premium contribution" is, from an economist's viewpoint, a tax, it is a well-disguised tax.) The Carter administration estimated that its Phase I National Health Plan would raise federal spending and total national spending by some $18 billion in 1980.

Such a plan is not necessarily incompatible with the procompetitive steps outlined in Chapter 8. In fact, the Carter plan includes requirements that employers offer all federally qualified HMOs in the areas where their employees live and that they contribute equally on behalf of insured plans and HMOs.

However, the basic flaw in this approach is that it accepts the present system with its perverse cost-increasing incentives pretty much as given. Fundamental delivery-system reform is not one of its design principles. Cost control would be left to public utility–type controls of the sort that have so far proved ineffective. Thus, for example, the system as proposed by Carter would include hospital-cost containment, health planning and certificate of need, a national limit on capital spending by hospitals (and hence political control), PSROs, and government-controlled physician fee schedules.

HealthCare, paying about 38 percent of the total costs of covered services, would be basically a fee-for-service cost-reimbursement system. The plan includes an HMO option for Medicare beneficiaries like the one described in Chapter 8.

Discussion

The Nixon and Carter plans would reinforce the link between jobs and health insurance. That is, health plans would continue to be tailored to the needs of specific employee groups rather than be designed to serve members of the community at large. And an employee's health plan coverage would continue to be tied to his or her job. The negative consequences of the job-related system of health insurance, described in Chapter 7, would continue.

I believe that reinforcing the link between jobs and health insurance is the wrong way to go. Instead, we should be moving away from a job-centered and toward a consumer-centered system of health insurance.

The Nixon and Carter plans do not create fair competition among health plans. They leave insurers free to experience rate their health insurance premiums. Thus employers of preferred-risk groups would continue to seek to lower their costs by offering an experience-rated insurance plan. This would leave the high-risk groups to be cared for by HMOs, which must practice community rating. Such a system leaves the market fragmented among groups of different risk classes.

There are other problems. A mandated premium contribution can act as an increase in the minimum wage and as a disincentive to hiring people of low productivity. However, the Carter plan mitigates this by limiting the employer's liability to 5 percent of payroll and subsidizing excess costs above that. Continuity of coverage provisions can be extremely costly in industries with higher turnover. The Carter administration estimated $450 per year as the cost of a family policy meeting minimum standards. That would come to about 23 cents per hour for a full-time employee. But if employers must continue coverage for at least ninety days after termination, that could mean 46 cents per hour for employers whose employees average three months—as in seasonal jobs. Again, presumably the limit on employer's cost of 5 percent of payroll would mitigate this problem.

GOVERNMENT AS UNIVERSAL THIRD-PARTY PAYOR

The third model of national health insurance is the government as universal third-party payor. The general idea is that if practically all health insurance is simply third-party payment of bills submitted by physicians and hospitals, the whole job of claims processing can be done far better and cheaper by a single agency. This might be a government agency, or it might be a private company on contract to the government. There are large economies of scale in computer processing, and there could be great economies from uniformity in claims forms. Doctors and hospitals would simply bill one payment agency instead of many. If eligibility for such a system were universal, many of the administrative complexities we face today would disappear. Providers would no longer have to determine how and whether each patient is insured. Their problems of collecting bills would disappear, as would all of the complexities of the link between jobs and health insurance.

Indeed, if today's dominant methods of payment—fee for service and cost reimbursement or cost-based charges—were inevitable, the case for such a system would be overwhelming. The whole case against it is based on the possibility of and need for fundamental delivery-system reform and a replacement of these forms of payment with alternative forms that produce more rational incentives.

One might characterize such a system as "Medicare for everybody." Universal health insurance on this model was proposed in 1974 by Senator Edward M. Kennedy and Ways and Means Committee Chairman Wilbur Mills, as mentioned above. Under that proposal, everybody would have been eligible for a comprehensive set of covered services, similar to those covered by Medicare, subject to an annual deductible of $150 per person, 25 percent coinsurance, and an annual maximum on cost sharing of $1000 per family. Cost sharing would have been reduced or eliminated for low-income families. The same model was adopted in Canada, for hospital services in 1957, and for physician services in 1968, with virtually no copayments or deductibles.

The shortcomings of the fee-for-service, cost-reimbursement, casualty-insurance system have been amply explained in this book, so there is no need to restate them. Let it suffice to note that by making this system universal, one would intensify the cost-increasing effect of the incentives contained in it. Thus such a system could be only transitional. Strong public utility–type controls would be needed to restrain costs.

But if such a system were in place, the government would inevitably notice, as it did in Canada, that it was paying thousands of hospital bills. Instead of paying them piecemeal, it would make more sense to negotiate a "global budget" with each hospital. At that point, every hospital would become completely dependent on government. There would be no need for certificate of need or hospital-cost containment. The industry would, in effect, be nationalized.

A similar process would occur with physician fees. The government would negotiate a fee schedule with the medical profession. Because of a lack of objective standards for determining what fees should be, the schedule would initially be what fees are now, modified to eliminate some of the most obvious inequities. Government would seek to control costs by holding the growth in fees to a rate below that of general inflation. This is what happened in Canada. One way of doing this has been simply to drag out negotiations and fail to agree on a new schedule. Doctors would seek to protect their real incomes by increasing the number and complexity of services performed, as described in Chapter 6. This process could not go on forever, however. I believe that the likely end-point of this process in Canada will be to move to something like the British system, in which hospital-based specialists are on salary, and community-based primary-care physicians are paid on a per capita basis for the number of people who sign up with them.

There is no doubt but that the growth in total spending can be controlled in such a system. Efficiency in the production of services and consumer satisfaction is another matter.

The worst effect of universal third-party payment by government is that it would destroy the incentives of consumers and physicians to form and join alternative delivery systems with built-in incentives for economy and consumer satisfaction. It would deny consumers the opportunity to realize the benefit from choosing less costly systems or styles of care; as in Medicare, larger reimbursements would be made on their behalf if they chose the more costly providers who ordered more tests, hospitalized more, and so forth. Similarly, with government-financed open-ended demand for services where and when they want to deliver them, physicians would see little gain from accepting the discipline of an organized system.

Prior to Canada's national health insurance, there had been a few attempts to start prepaid group practices there, but they faced intense opposition from the medical profession. In effect, the arrival of national health insurance in Canada put them out of business as capitation-financed enterprises. The government could deal with them only on a budget-and-salary basis or a fee-for-service basis. Eugene Vayda, M.D., of the Department of Health Administration, University of Toronto, summarized the experience as follows:

> In order to plan and budget for medical services a prepaid health plan must be able to enroll members and limit their out-of-plan use by not paying for it. Provincial governments have not been willing to adopt enrollment or to deny insurance coverage for out-of-plan utilization. Denial of payment for any health care services is seen as incompatible with universal insurance. . . . The prospects for group practice in . . . Canada are reasonable, but capitation prepaid group practice programs, particularly new ones, face a bleak future.
>
> Wherever adopted, universal health insurance has tended to fix the existing health care system and its payment mechanisms. This was the case in Canada. Prepaid group practice was in a weak bargaining position at the time of universal medical insurance. . . . Unless ways are developed to deal with the problems of enrollment, opposition and capitalization, prepaid group practice may never become a factor in Canadian health care delivery.[9]

NOTES

CHAPTER 1

1. Kenneth J. Arrow, "Uncertainty and the Welfare Economics of Medical Care," *American Economic Review* **53** (1963): 941-1973.
2. Walter McClure, "Memorandum I: Essential Points to Understanding the Major Options Available in National Health Insurance," Excelsior, MN: Inter-Study, August 20, 1974.
3. John P. Gilbert, Richard J. Light, and Frederick Mosteller, "Assessing Social Innovations: An Empirical Base for Policy," in *Evaluation and Experiment: Some Critical Issues in Assessing Social Programs*, ed. Carl A. Bennett and Arthur A. Lumsdaine, New York: Academic Press, 1975.
4. Benjamin A. Barnes, "Discarded Operations: Surgical Innovation by Trial and Error," in *Costs, Risks, and Benefits of Surgery*, ed. John P. Bunker, Benjamin A. Barnes, and Frederick Mosteller, New York: Oxford University Press, 1977.
5. Lillian Lin Miao, "Gastric Freezing: An Example of the Evaluation of Medical Therapy by Randomized Clinical Trials," in *Costs, Risks, and Benefits of Surgery, op. cit.*; Ernest M. Barsamian, "The Rise and Fall of Internal Mammary Artery Ligation in the Treatment of Angina-Pectoris and the Lessons Learned," in *Costs, Risks, and Benefits of Surgery, op. cit.*
6. H. G. Mather *et al.*, "Acute Myocardial Infarction: Home and Hospital Treatment," in *British Medical Journal*, (1971): 334-338.
7. A. L. Cochrane, *Effectiveness and Efficiency: Random Reflections on Health Services*, London: Burgess & Son (Abingdon) Ltd. for The Nuffield Provincial Hospital Trust, 1972.
8. J. D. Hill, J. R. Hampton, and J. R. A. Mitchell, "A Randomized Trial of Home versus Hospital Management for Patients with Suspected Myocardial Infarction," *The Lancet* (April 22, 1978): 837-841.
9. Joseph Newhouse and Lindy J. Friedlander, *The Relationship Between Medical Resources and Measures of Health: Some Additional Evidence*, Santa Monica, CA: The RAND Corporation, R-2066-HEW, May 1977.
10. Michael K. Miller and C. Shannon Stokes, "Health Status, Health Resources, and Consolidated Structural Parameters: Implications for Public Health Care Policy," *Journal of Health and Social Behavior* **19** (September 1978): 263-279.
11. Paul A. Lembcke, "Measuring the Quality of Medical Care Through Vital Statistics Based on Hospital Service Areas: 1. Comparative Study of Appendectomy Rates," *American Journal of Public Health* **42** (March 1952): 276-286.
12. S. Lichtner and M. Pflanz, "Appendectomy in the Federal Republic of Germany: Epidemiology and Medical Care Patterns," *Medical Care*, 9 (1971): 311.
13. Milton Silverman and Philip R. Lee, *Pills, Profits and Politics*, Berkeley: University of California Press, 1974.
14. Anne A. Scitovsky and Nelda M. Snyder, "Effects of Coinsurance on Use of Physician Services," *Social Security Bulletin* **35,** 6 (June 1972): 3-19.
15. George N. Monsma, Jr., "Marginal Revenue and the Demand for Physicians' Services," in *Empirical Studies in Health Economics*, ed. Herbert E. Klarman, Baltimore: Johns Hopkins University Press, 1970.

16. Harold S. Luft, "How Do Health-Maintenance Organizations Achieve Their 'Savings'?" *New England Journal of Medicine* **298** (June 15, 1978): 1336–1343.

CHAPTER 2

1. Robert M. Gibson, "National Health Expenditures, 1978," *Health Care Financing Review* **1** (Summer 1979): 1–36.
2. Martin S. Feldstein and Amy Taylor, *The Rapid Rise of Hospital Costs*, Washington, D.C.: staff report, Council on Wage and Price Stability, January 1977.
3. Marjorie Smith Mueller, "Private Health Insurance in 1975; Coverage, Enrollment, and Financial Experience," *Social Security Bulletin* **40** (June 1977): 3–21.
4. "Profile of Health-Care Coverage: The Haves and Have-Nots," background paper, Washington, D.C.: Congressional Budget Office, March 1979.
5. Feldstein and Taylor, *op. cit.*
6. Eugene Steuerle and Ronald Hoffman, "Tax Expenditures for Health Care," OTA Paper No. 38. Washington, D.C.: Office of Tax Analysis, Assistant Secretary for Tax Policy, Department of Treasury, April 1979.
7. Mark S. Blumberg, "Rational Provider Prices: Provider Price Changes for Improved Health Care Use," in *Health Handbook*, ed. George K. Chacko, Amsterdam: North Holland Publishing Co., 1979.
8. Reuben A. Kessel, "Price Discrimination in Medicine," *Journal of Law and Economics* **1** (October 1958): 20–53.
9. Blumberg, *op. cit.*
10. Stephen J. Dresnick et al., "The Physician's Role in the Cost-Containment Problem," *Journal of the American Medical Association* **241** (April 1979): 1606–1609; also, James K. Skipper et al., "Physician's Knowledge of Cost: The Case of Diagnostic Tests," *Inquiry* **13** (June 1976): 194–198.
11. Harold A. Cohen, "Evaluating the Cost of Technology," in *Technology and the Cost of Health Care*, hearings before the Subcommittee on Domestic and International Scientific Planning, Analysis, and Cooperation, Washington, D.C.: Government Printing Office, 36-163-0, 1979.
12. Victor R. Fuchs and Marcia J. Kramer, *Determinants of Expenditures for Physicians' Services in the United States, 1948–68*, New York: National Bureau of Economic Research, 1973.
13. Frank A. Sloan and Roger Feldman, "Competition Among Physicians," in *Competition in the Health Care Sector, Past, Present, and Future*, ed. Warren Greenberg. Proceedings of a conference sponsored by the Bureau of Economics, Federal Trade Commission, March 1978, Germantown, MD: Aspen Systems Corp. 1978; Uwe E. Reinhardt, "Comment," in *Competition in the Health Care Sector: Past, Present, and Future, op. cit.*; Joseph P. Newhouse, *The Economics of Medical Care*, Reading, MA: Addison-Wesley, 1978; Jerry Green, "Physician-Induced Demand for Medical Care," *Journal of Human Resources*, **13** Supplement 1978: 21–34.
14. Victor R. Fuchs, "The Supply of Surgeons and the Demand for Operations," *Journal of Human Resources* **13** Supplement 1978: 35–56.
15. Uwe E. Reinhardt, *Physician Productivity and the Demand for Health Manpower*, Cambridge, MA: Ballinger Publishing Company, 1975.

16. *Assessing the Efficacy and Safety of Medical Technology,* Washington, D.C.: Office of Technology Assessment, September 1978.

17. Louise B. Russell, "The Diffusion of New Hospital Technologies in the United States," *International Journal of Health Services* **6,** 4 (1976): 557–580.

18. *Development of Medical Technology Opportunities for Assessment,* Washington, D.C.: Office of Technology Assessment, August 1976.

19. *Policy Implications of the Computed Tomography (CT) Scanner,* Washington, D.C.: Office of Technology Assessment, August 1978.

20. Richard Rettig, "End-Stage Renal Disease and the 'Cost' of Medical Technology," in *Medical Technology: The Culprit Behind Health Care Costs?* ed. Stuart H. Altman and Robert Blendon, Washington, D.C.: Department of Health, Education, and Welfare, Publication No. (PHS) 79-3216, 1979, pp. 88–115.

21. Martin S. Feldstein, "A New Approach to National Health Insurance," *The Public Interest* (Spring 1971): 93–105 and "The High Cost of Hospitals—and What to Do About It," *The Public Interest* (Summer 1977): 40–54.

22. Laurence S. Seidman, "Supplementary Health Insurance and Cost-Consciousness Strategy," *Journal of Risk and Insurance* **45,** 2 (June 1978): 291–310.

CHAPTER 3

1. Steven A. Finkler, "Cost Effectiveness of Regionalization: The Heart Surgery Example," *Inquiry* **16,** 3 (Fall 1979): 264–270. See also, Maurice McGregor and Gerald Pelletier, "Planning of Specialized Health Facilities, Size vs. Cost and Effectiveness in Heart Surgery," *New England Journal of Medicine* **299** (July 27, 1978): 179–181.

2. Harold S. Luft, John P. Bunker, and Alain C. Enthoven, "Should Operations Be Regionalized? The Empirical Relation Between Surgical Volume and Mortality," *New England Journal of Medicine* **301,** 25 (December 20, 1979): 1364–1369.

3. Ann H. Pettigrew, "Final Report of the Massachusetts Maternity and Newborn Regionalization Project," Massachusetts Department of Public Health, August 1, 1974–September 30, 1976.

4. *Characteristics of Physicians,* Chicago: American Medical Association, December 31, 1975; *Physician Distribution and Medical Licensure in the U.S., 1977,* Chicago: American Medical Association, 1979; Kaiser-Permanente Medical Care Program.

5. Katherine K. Carter and Thaine H. Allison, Jr., *A Comparison of Utilization and Costs in Kaiser and Non-Kaiser Hospitals in California,* Research Report 78-2, California Health Facilities Commission, State of California, November 1978.

6. Alan M. Gittelsohn and John E. Wennberg, "On the Incidence of Tonsillectomy and Other Surgical Procedures," in *Costs, Risks, and Benefits of Surgery,* ed. John P. Bunker, Benjamin A. Barnes, and Frederick Mosteller, New York: Oxford University Press, 1977.

7. John E. Wennberg, "Getting Ready for National Health Insurance: Unnecessary Surgery," testimony and statement presented at the hearings before the Subcommittee on Oversight and Investigations of the Committee on Interstate and Foreign Commerce, House of Representatives, 94th Congress, July 15, 1975.

8. Adolph M. Hutter, Jr., *et al.*, "Early Hospital Discharge After Myocardial Infarction," *New England Journal of Medicine* **288,** 22 (May 31, 1973): 1141-1144.

9. *Ibid.*

10. J. Frederick McNeer *et al.*, "Hospital Discharge One Week After Acute Myocardial Infarction," *New England Journal of Medicine* **298,** 5 (February 2, 1978): 229-232.

11. Eugene G. McCarthy and Geraldine Widmer, "Effects of Screening by Consultants on Recommended Elective Surgical Procedures," *New England Journal of Medicine* **291,** 25 (December 19, 1974): 1331-1335; also, Eugene G. McCarthy, "Unnecessary Surgery," testimony presented at the hearings before the Subcommittee on Oversight and Investigations of the Committee on Interstate and Foreign Commerce, House of Representatives, 94th Congress, July 15, 17, 18, September 3, 1975.

12. John P. Bunker and B. William Brown, Jr., "The Physician-Patient as an Informed Consumer of Surgical Services," *New England Journal of Medicine* **290** (1974): 1051-1055.

13. *Assessing the Efficacy and Safety of Medical Technologies,* Washington, D.C.: Office of Technology Assessment, September 1978.

14. Raymond R. Neutra *et al.*, "Effect of Fetal Monitoring on Neonatal Death Rates," *New England Journal of Medicine* **299** (August 17, 1978): 324-326.

15. David M. Eddy, "Clinical Policies and the Quality of Clinical Practice," Parts I and II, Program for the Analysis of Clinical Policies, Stanford, CA: Stanford University, Department of Engineering and Economic Systems, Report 79-1, 1979.

16. David M. Eddy, *Rationale for the Cancer Screening Benefit Program: Screening Policies,* Stanford, CA: Stanford University, Departments of Family, Community, and Preventive Medicine and of Engineering-Economic Systems, for the Blue Cross Association, January 1978.

17. Benjamin A. Barnes, "Discarded Operations: Surgical Innovation by Trial and Error," in *Costs, Risks, and Benefits of Surgery, op. cit.*

18. John P. Gilbert, Buckman McPeek, and Frederick Mosteller, "Progress in Surgery and Anesthesia: Benefits and Risks of Innovative Therapy," in *Costs, Risks and Benefits of Surgery, op. cit.*; also, John P. Gilbert, Richard J. Light, and Frederick Mosteller, "Assessing Social Innovations: An Empirical Base for Policy," in *Evaluation and Experiment: Some Critical Issues in Assessing Social Programs,* ed. Carl A. Bennett and Arthur A. Lumsdaine, New York: Academic Press, 1975.

19. Marvin L. Murphy *et al.*, "Treatment of Chronic Stable Angina: A Preliminary Report of Survival Data of the Randomized Veterans Administration Cooperative Study," *New England Journal of Medicine* **297,** 12 (September 22, 1977): 621-627.

20. *Policy Implications of the Computed Tomography (CT) Scanner,* Washington, D.C.: Office of Technology Assessment, August 1978.

21. *Computed Tomographic Scanning,* Washington, D.C.: Institute of Medicine, National Academy of Sciences, 1977.

22. John P. Bunker, David Hinkley, and W. V. McDermott, "Surgical Innovation and Its Evaluation," *Science* **200** (May 26, 1978): 937-941.

23. Nancy H. Bryant, Louise Candland, and Regina Loewenstein, "Comparison of Care and Cost Outcomes for Stroke Patients with and without Home Care," *Stroke* **5** (January–February 1974): 54-59.

24. Duncan Robertson, R. Amos Griffiths, and Lionel Z. Cosin, "A Community-Based Continuing Care Program for the Elderly Disabled," *Journal of Gerontology* **32**, 3 (1977): 334–339; also, Philip W. Brickner *et al.*, "The Homebound Aged: A Medically Unreached Group, *Annals of Internal Medicine* **82**, 1 (1975): 1.

CHAPTER 4

1. Paul M. Ellwood *et al.*, "Health Maintenance Strategy," proposal first presented to the Secretary of Health, Education, and Welfare, March 1970, and subsequently published in *Medical Care* **291** (May 1971): 250–256.
2. Paul M. Ellwood and Walter McClure, *Health Delivery Reform*, Excelsior, MN: InterStudy, September 10, 1976 (revised November 17, 1976).
3. Walter McClure, "On Broadening the Definition of and Removing Regulatory Barriers of a Competitive Health Care System," *Journal of Health Politics, Policy and Law* **3**, 3 (Fall 1978): 303–327.
4. "National HMO Census of Prepaid Plans, 1978," Rockville, MD: Department of Health, Education, and Welfare, Office of Health Maintenance Organizations, Public Health Service, 1978.
5. Harold S. Luft, "How Do Health Maintenance Organizations Achieve Their 'Savings'?" *New England Journal of Medicine* **298**, 24 (June 15, 1978): 1336–1343.
6. Donald C. Riedel *et al.*, *Federal Employees' Health Benefits Program, Utilization Study*, Rockville, MD: Department of Health, Education, and Welfare, National Center for Health Services Research, Health Resources Administration, Publication No. (HRA) 75-3125, January 1975.
7. Mildred Corbin and Aaron Krute, "Some Aspects of Medicare Experience with Group-Practice Prepayment Plans," *Social Security Bulletin* **38**, 3 (March 1975): 3–11; also, Steve Goss, *A Retrospective Application of the Health Maintenance Organization Risk-Sharing Savings Formula for Six Group Practice Prepayment Plans for 1969 and 1970*, Washington, D.C.: Actuarial Note No. 88, DHEW Publication No. (SSA) 76-11500, 1975.
8. Paul M. Ellwood, "Health Delivery in Transition," statement before the Congress of the United States, House of Representatives, Subcommittee on Health and Environment, Washington, D.C.: February 10, 1976; also, Anne A. Scitovsky and Nelda McCall, "Use of Hospital Services under Two Prepaid Plans," *Medical Care* **18**, 1 (January 1980).
9. "The Doctors and HMO's: An Analysis," *Medical World News* **19**, 5 (March 6, 1978): 81.
10. Luft, *op. cit.*
11. Richard H. Egdahl *et al.*, "The Potential of Organizations of Fee-for-Service Physicians for Achieving Significant Decreases in Hospitalization," *Annals of Surgery* **186**, 3 (September 1977): 388–399.
12. Stephen Moore, "Cost Containment Through Risk-Sharing by Primary-Care Physicians," *New England Journal of Medicine* **300**, 24 (June 14, 1979): 1359–1362.
13. Robert E. Schlenker *et al.*, *HMOs in 1973, A National Survey*. Excelsior, MN: InterStudy, February 1974; also, "National HMO Census of Prepaid Plans, 1978," *op. cit.*

CHAPTER 5

1. Charles L. Schultze, *The Public Use of Private Interest*, Washington, D.C.: Brookings Institution, 1977.
2. Mildred Corbin and Aaron Krute, "Some Aspects of Medicare Experience with Group-Practice Prepayment Plans," *Social Security Bulletin* **38**, 3 (March 1975): pp. 3-11; also in Steve Goss, "A Retrospective Application of the Health Maintenance Organization Risk-Sharing Savings Formula for Six Group Practice Prepayment Plans for 1969 and 1970," Washington, D.C.: Department of Health, Education, and Welfare, Actuarial Note No. 88, Publication No. (SSA) 76-11500, 1975.
3. William Hsiao, "Public versus Private Administration of Health Insurance: A Study in Relative Economic Efficiency," *Inquiry* **15**, 4 (December 1978): 379-387.
4. Andrew E. Ruddock, "Federal Employees Health Benefits Program. I. History and Future of the Federal Program—1964," *American Journal of Public Health* **56**, 1 (1966): 50-53. Reprinted by permission.
5. Jon B. Christianson, *Do HMOs Stimulate Beneficial Competition?*, Excelsior, MN: InterStudy, April 27, 1978.
6. Edmund Faltermayer, "Where Doctors Scramble for Patients' Dollars," *Fortune*, November 6, 1978, pp. 114-120.
7. Jon B. Christianson and Walter McClure, "Competition in the Delivery of Medical Care," *New England Journal of Medicine* **301**, 15 (October 11, 1979): 812-818.
8. *Health Care Trends: Minneapolis/St. Paul, Summary Highlights*, Excelsior, MN: InterStudy, August 1979; also, *Report of the 1978 Annual Survey*, Chicago: American Hospital Association, Office of Policy Studies, Policy Brief No. 18, 1979.

CHAPTER 6

1. Alain C. Enthoven and Roger G. Noll, "Regulatory and Non-Regulatory Strategies for Controlling Health Care Costs," in *Medical Technology: The Culprit Behind Health Care Costs?* ed. Stuart Altman and Robert Blendon, Washington, D.C.: Department of Health, Education, and Welfare, Publication No. (PHS) 79-3216, 1979.
2. *Ibid.*
3. Paul B. Ginsburg, "Inflation and the Economic Stabilization Program," in *Health: A Victim or Cause of Inflation?* ed. Michael Zubkoff, New York: Prodist, 1976.
4. Paul B. Ginsburg, "Impact of the Economic Stabilization Program on Hospitals: An Analysis with Aggregate Data," in *Hospital Cost Containment Selected Notes for Future Policy*, ed. Michael Zubkoff, Ira E. Raskin, and Ruth S. Hanft, New York: Prodist, 1978.
5. *Ibid.*

6. Frank A. Sloan and Bruce Steinwald, "Effects of Regulation on Hospital Costs and Input Use," *Journal of Law and Economics* (forthcoming).

7. *Controlling Rising Hospital Costs*, Washington, D.C.: Congressional Budget Office, September 1979.

8. Harold A. Cohen, "Experience of a State Cost Control Commission," in *Hospital Cost Containment: Selected Notes for Future Policy, op. cit.*

9. "Evaluation of the Efficiency and Effectiveness of the Section 1122 Review Process," Washington, D.C.: Lewin & Associates, September 1975.

10. David S. Salkever and Thomas W. Bice, "The Impact of Certificate-of-Need Controls on Hospital Investment," *Health and Society, Milbank Memorial Fund Quarterly* **54,** 2 (Spring 1976): 185–214.

11. Fred J. Hellinger, "The Effect of Certificate-of-Need Legislation on Hospital Investment," *Inquiry* **13,** 2 (June 1976): 187–193.

12. Frank A. Sloan and Bruce Steinwald, *op. cit.*

13. *A Policy Statement: Controlling the Supply of Hospital Beds*, Washington, D.C.: Institute of Medicine, National Academy of Sciences, October 1976.

14. "Certificate-of-Need Application No. 78-036 for Open-Heart Surgery Unit," Oakland, CA: Kaiser-Permanente Medical Center, April 13, 1978.

15. Staff Analysis; Dan Feshban, principal author, "Kaiser-Permanente Medical Center Certificate-of-Need Application No. 78-036 for Open-Heart Surgery Unit," San Francisco: West Bay Health Systems Agency, August 25, 1978.

16. Nancy L. Worthington, "National Health Expenditures, 1929–1974," *Social Security Bulletin* **38,** 2 (February 1975): pp. 3–20.

17. Zachary Y. Dyckman, *A Study of Physicians' Fees*, Washington, D.C.: Council on Wage and Price Stability, Executive Office of the President, March 1978.

18. Robert G. Evans, "Beyond the Medical Market Place: Expenditure, Utilization and Pricing of Insured Health in Canada," in *National Health Insurance: Can We Learn from Canada?* ed. Spyros Andreopoulos, New York: Wiley, 1975.

19. Social Security Amendments of 1972: Report of the Committee on Finance, United States Senate, to Accompany H.R.1, to Amend the Social Security Act and for Other Purposes, 92nd Congress, Second Session, Senate Report No. 92-1230, 9/26/1972, pp. 254–255.

20. *Ibid.*

21. Clark C. Havighurst and James F. Blumstein, "Coping with Quality/Cost Trade-Offs in Medical Care: The Role of PSROs," *Northwestern University Law Review* **70,** 1 (March–April 1975): 6–68.

22. Robert H. Brook, Kathleen N. Williams, and John E. Rolph, with the assistance of Bryant Mori, *Controlling the Use and Cost of Medical Services: the New Mexico Experimental Medical Care Review Organization—A Four-Year Case Study*, Santa Monica, CA: RAND Corporation, Publ. R-2241-HEW, November 1978.

23. *Ibid.*

24. Paul B. Ginsburg and Daniel M. Koretz, *The Effect of PSROs on Health Care Costs: Current Findings and Future Evaluations*, Washington, D.C.: Congressional Budget Office, June 1979; Health Care Financing Administration, *Professional Standards Review Organization 1978 Program Evaluation*, Washington, D.C.: U.S. Department of Health, Education, and Welfare, H.E.W. Publication No. HCFA-03000, January 1979.

25. Thomas G. Moore, "Deregulating Surface Freight Transportation," in *Promoting Competition In Regulated Markets*, ed. Almarin Phillips, Washington, D.C.: The Brookings Institution, 1975.

26. Roger G. Noll, "The Consequences of Public Utility Regulation of Hospitals," reproduced from *Controls on Health Care,* pp. 25-48, with the permission of the Institute of Medicine, National Academy of Sciences, Washington, D.C., 1975.
27. Charles L. Schultze, *The Public Use of Private Interest,* Washington, D.C.: The Brookings Institution, 1977.

CHAPTER 7

1. Odin W. Anderson and J. Joel May, "The Federal Employees Health Benefits Program, 1961-1968; A Model for National Health Insurance?" in *A9 Perspectives,* Chicago: Center for Health Administration Studies, University of Chicago, 1971.
2. Herman M. Somers and Anne R. Somers, "Major Issues in National Health Insurance," *Milbank Memorial Fund Quarterly* **50** (April 1972): 177-210.
3. Walter J. McNerney, statement on national health insurance presented before the Subcommittee on Health, Committee on Ways and Means, Washington, D.C.: April 15, 1975.
4. Alain C. Enthoven, memorandum for Secretary of HEW Joseph Califano, on national health insurance, September 22, 1977; also, ———, "Consumer Choice Health Plan" (in two parts), *New England Journal of Medicine* **298** (March 23 and 30, 1978): 650-658 and 709-720.
5. Alain C. Enthoven, "Consumer-Centered vs. Job-Centered Health Insurance," *Harvard Business Review* **57,** 1 (January–February 1979): 141-152.
6. Karen Davis, "Equal Treatment and Unequal Benefits: The Medicare Program," *Health and Society,* New York: Milbank Memorial Fund, Fall 1975.
7. Eugene Steuerle and Ronald Hoffman, *Tax Expenditures for Health Care,* Washington, D.C.: Department of the Treasury, Office of Tax Analysis (OTA Paper No. 38), April 1979.
8. *Can Health Maintenance Organizations Be Successful? An Analysis of 14 Federally Qualified HMOs,* Report to the Congress of the United States, Washington, D.C.: The Comptroller General, HRD-78-125, June 30, 1978.
9. *Ibid.*

CHAPTER 8

1. Address by The Honorable Al Ullman, Chairman, Committee on Ways and Means, at the *National Journal* Conference on Health Policy, Washington, D.C.: June 7, 1979.
2. *Ibid.*
3. Health Cost Restraint Act of 1979, H.R. 5740, 96th Congress, 1st Session, October 30, 1979.
4. Health Incentives Reform Act of 1979, S.1485, 96th Congress of the United States, 1st session, July 12, 1979.
5. *Congressional Record,* Washington, D.C.: United States Senate, June 12, 1979.

6. Dave Stockman, "Rethinking Federal Health Policy: Unshackle the Health Care Consumer," reprinted by permission from the *National Journal, the Washington Weekly on Government Affairs* **11** (June 2, 1979): 934–936.
7. John Maynard Keynes, *The General Theory of Employment, Interest and Money,* New York: Harcourt, Brace & Co., 1935.
8. *Ibid.*

APPENDIX

1. Saul Waldman, comp. *National Health Insurance Proposals Provisions of Bills Introduced in the 94th Congress as of February 1976,* Washington, D.C., Department of Health, Education, and Welfare, Office of Research and Statistics, Publication No. (SSA) 76-11920, March 1976.
2. S.4297, 91st Congress, Second Session, August 27, 1970.
3. S.3286, 93rd Congress, Second Session, April 2, 1974.
4. S.1720, 96th Congress, First Session, September 6, 1979; see also "Health Care for All Americans" and "Detailed Explanation of Health Care for All Americans Plan," distributed by Senator Kennedy's office, May 14, 1979.
5. *Health Care for American Veterans,* Report of the Committee on Health-care Resources in the Veterans Administration, Assembly of Life Sciences, Washington, D.C.: National Research Council/National Academy of Sciences, May 1977.
6. *Report of the Military Health Care Study, Supplement: Detailed Findings,* Washington, D.C.: Department of Defense; Department of Health, Education, and Welfare; and Office of Management and Budget, USGPO 041-014-00037-7, December 1975.
7. S.2970, 93rd Congress, Second Session, February 6, 1974.
8. *President Carter's National Health Plan Legislation,* Summary Fact Sheet and Detailed Fact Sheet, Washington, D.C.: The White House, June 12, 1979. Also, the National Health Plan Act, S.1812, 96th Congress, 1st Session, September 25, 1979.
9. Eugene Vayda, "Prepaid Group Practice Under Universal Health Insurance in Canada," *Medical Care* **15,** 5 (May 1977): 382–389.

INDEX

INDEX

A

Actuarial costs, determining, 120
Adjusted average per capita cost, 124
Administrative services only (ASO)
    contracts, 26
Alcoholism, 15
Aliens, illegal, financing health care
    for, 131–132
Allowable costs, 24
American Medical Association, and
    Federal Trade Commission
    suit, 27
Anderson, Odin, 114
Angina pectoris, 3, 5. *See also* Heart
    attack patients
Antibiotics, excessive, 8
Appendectomy, per capita rate of, 7
Arrow, Kenneth, 2
Arson, commercial, 11
Art, medical care as, 9

B

Barnes, Benjamin, 4
"Basic health services," 127–128
Benefit-cost analysis, need for, 49–50.
    See also Costs
Benefit plans. *See also* Health plans
    cafeteria-style, 148
    control over, 74, 155
    standards for, 149–150
Benefits, health
    and law of diminishing marginal
        returns, 45
    100 percent employer-paid, 20
    political significance of, 19
    and "swiss cheese policies," 124
Bice, Thomas, 102
Biopsies, 2

Blue Cross–Blue Shield plans
    and alternative delivery systems,
        xxiv, 155
    and antitrust suits, 134
    and CCHP, 144
    in CCHP transition, 132–133
    and FEHBP, 115
    and inpatient routine testing, 54
    in Kennedy health plan, 162
    as option for federal employees, 82
    in Pennsylvania, 64
    as third-party payor, 16
    in Washington, D.C., study, 59
Blumberg, Mark, 21
Brown, Byron, Jr., 47
Bunker, John, 39, 41, 47, 53

C

Caesarian sections, increase in, 48
Califano, Joseph, 115
California, physician supply in, 43
Canada, national health insurance
    system in, 107, 171–172
Caring, vs. curing, 5. *See also* Medical
    care
Carter administration, 97–98, 100,
    105, 147
    health plan proposal of, 115, 168–
        170
    welfare-reform proposal of, 123
Casualty insurance model, of health
    care financing, 1, 155
    failure of, 8
    limitations of, xviii, 10–12
Catastrophic expense protection, 129,
    149
Catastrophic health insurance, 157
C.A.T. scanning, 29–30, 52–53
Certificate-of-need (CON) laws, xx,
    101–105

Charges, "customary and
    prevailing," 26. *See also* Fee
    structure
Choicecare, 62
Christianson, Jon, 88
Chrysler, health insurance costs of,
    xv
Civilian Health and Medical Program
    of the Uniformed Services
    (CHAMPUS), 131
Civil Service Commission, 143, 144
Claims processing, costs of, 83
Clinical trials, 51–52
Cochrane, A. L., 6
Cohen, Harold A., 101
Coinsurance
    reliance on, 34
    unworkability of, 32–36
Community rating, 127
    defined, 80
    required, 94–95, 150
Competition, economic
    desirability of, 57
    explanation of, 72–73
    between Hawaii's health plans, 85
    among health plans, 20
    among HMOs, 86–87, 91
    and information costs, 81
    under Kennedy plan, 164–165
    under Nixon and Carter plans, 170
    prepaid group practices in, 92
    principles of, 71–72
    vs. regulation, xx, xxi–xxii, 93–95
    socially desirable, 126
Comprecare, 62
Comprehensive Health Care
    Program, Pennsylvania Blue
    Shield's, 64
Comprehensive Health Insurance Act
    of 1974, 158, 167–170
Computerized axial tomography, 29–
    30, 52–53
Congress, and delivery system
    reform, 151–153. *See also*
    National health insurance
Congressional Budget Office, 17
Consumer Choice Health Plan
    (CCHP), xxiii, 154
    alternatives to, 157

background of, 114
criticism of, 137
description of, 115–119
and fairness to poor, 139
and federal budget, 134–137
and federal-state roles, 130
and FEHBP, 119
financing of, 119–126, 134–137
problems with, 142–144
reorganization under, 137–138
results of, 140–142
and socially desirable competition,
    127
transition period for, 132–133
and underserved rural areas, 140
Consumer price index (CPI), and
    physicians' fees, 106
Consumers. *See also* Patients
    and CCHP, 138–139
    choices for, 145–146
    cost consciousness of, 35, 36
    and impact of regulatory practices,
        112
    and increase in insurance
        premiums, 18–19
    lack of multiple choice for, 73–75
    multiple choice for, 71
    and quality of care, 60
Continuity of coverage, as required
    standard, 149–150
"Cookbook medicine," 4
Copayments
    under Canadian system, 171
    under Carter plan, 168
    as consumer control, 129
Coronary artery bypass graft surgery,
    5, 52
Coronary care units (CCUs), 6, 7
Cost consciousness, 53–54
Cost controls, government vs. self-
    imposed, 63
"Cost-effectiveness"
    analysis, 49–50, 165–166
    CCHP incentives for, 137
Cost efficiency, and volume of
    operations, 38
Cost overruns, estimating, 135
Costs
    actuarial, 120

adjusted average per capita, 124
allowable, 24
information, 81
of Kennedy health plan, 166
in prepaid group practices, 58
routine, 24
total vs. premium, 59
Costs, hospital
and CON controls, 102–104
containment of, 95–101
and HMOs, xxiii
measuring increase in, 96
and price-control programs, 97
reasonableness of, 26
reimbursement for, 24–25
Costs, medical
and aging population, 31
attempts to control, 32
in CCHP, 141
and "defensive" medicine, 32
impact of HMOs on, 88
and IPAs, 63
physicians' control of, 23
and prepaid groups, 60
prepaid group practices vs.
Medicare, 76
and price-control programs, 97
and primary care networks, 65–66
regional differences in, 28
and technological advances, 30
uncertainty of, 11, 34

D

Death rates, neonatal, 49
Deductibles
under Canadian system, 171
under Carter plan, 168
as consumer control, 129
unworkability of, 32–36
Defense Department, health care
system of, xxi, 131–132, 160
Delivery systems
alternative, xix, xxiv, 56, 155
competition afforded by, 69
fair economic competition of, 78,
89–92
growth of, 67, 91

individual practice associations,
61
prepaid group practice, 57–61
primary care networks, 64–66
reform, 91, 118, 133–134
Demand, doctor-created, 27–28
Dermatology, physician supply in, 43
Diagnostic tests
duplicate, 54
reliability of, 2
and technological advances, 30
Dialysis
home, 30
renal, 29
Diminishing marginal returns, law
of, 45–46
Disease, physician-caused
(iatrogenic), 7
Doctors. *See also* Physicians
benefits of limited choice of, 56
in CCHP, 140
in competing economic units, 72
disagreement among, 3
free choice and cost control, xviii
free choice vs. cost-containment
incentives, 56
geographic distribution of, xvii, 43
hospital competition for, 23
insurance coverage with free choice
of, 23
Doctor visits
compressibility of, 107
unnecessary, 31–32
Drug reactions, adverse, 8
Durenberger, David, 152, 156
Dyckman, Zachary, 106

E

Economic Stabilization Program, xx,
95, 105–106
Economy
fair competition in, 71 (*see also*
Competition)
free-market, 70
and health care quality, xix
Eddy, David, 49

Elderly
  increase in numbers of, 31
  private insurance for, 18
Eligibility, Medicaid, 18
Ellwood, Paul, 23, 55, 56
Employees
  choice offered to, xxiii
  health care incentives for, 20
Employers
  choices offered to employees, 145–
    148
  and costs of health insurance, 59
  equal fixed-dollar contributions of,
    148
  and health benefits, 19 (*see also*
    Benefits)
  and HMOs, 86–87
  insurance offered by, xvi, 73, 75
  under Kennedy plan, 162
  nonprofit, 146
  packages negotiated by, 117
  tax-free contributions of, 150
Enrollment process
  and fair economic competition, 127
  government supervision of, 119
Evans, Robert, 107
Executive pay, politics of, 161
Expectations, and demand for health
    care services, 15
Expenditures, health. *See also*
    Spending
  national, 13 (*see also* National
    health insurance)
  physicians' control of, 118
  real per capita, 14
  regional differences in, 126
"Experience effect," 39–40
Experience rating, 25, 80, 116, 153

F

Facilities
  excess, 60
  matching with needs, 44
"False-positive rate," 49
Federal Aviation Administration, 93–
    95

Federal Employees' Health Benefits
    Program (FEHBP), xxii, xxiii, 79
  description of, 82–84
  and political influences, 143
Federal government. *See also*
    Legislation
  and CCHP costs, 134–137
  and CCHP financing and
    administration, 130
  and health care spending, 14, 15
  as third-party payor, 25, 158, 170–
    172
Federal Trade Commission, and
    unfair health trade practices,
    134
Fee-for-service system, xviii, 21–23,
    42–44
  alternative to, 57
  and defined population, 57
  disadvantages of, xvi-xvii
  excess costs in, 60
  fair economic competition in, 90
  and hospital use, 61
  and Medicare reform, 125
  vs. prepaid group practice, 59
  retainer, 23
  subsidies provided for, 77
Fee structure. *See also* Physicians' fees
  and hospitalization, 22
  usual, customary, and reasonable
    (UCR), 105
Feldstein, Martin, 18, 32
Fetal monitoring, electronic, cost
    containment in, 48–49
Financing health care. *See also* Health
    plans
  alternative plans for, xix, xxiv
  casualty insurance model for, xviii,
    1, 8, 10–12, 155
  free choice of doctor in, 77
  public-utility approach to, 5
Finkler, Steven, 37, 38, 39
Fixed-dollar subsidies, principle of,
    xxii
Fleming, Scott, 114
Foreign medical graduates, 27
Free choice of doctor, xviii
  and insurance coverage, 26
  and Medicare reform, 125

Free-market system, 70
Fuchs, Victor, 27, 42

G

General Accounting Office (GAO),
    HMO evaluation of, 143
General Motors, health insurance
    costs of, xv
Georgetown University Community
    Health Plan, 58, 61
Gilmore, Martha, 75
Ginsburg, Paul, 96, 98, 109
Gittelsohn, Alan, 46
Government, as insurer, 26. *See also*
    Federal government; State
    government
Gross national product, health care
    spending in, 13
Group Health Association, of
    Washington, D.C., 58
Group Health Cooperative (Puget
    Sound), 44, 58, 65, 68, 124
Group Health Plan (Minnesota), 86
Group Health Plan of Northeast
    Ohio, 64
Group practices
    multispecialty, 59
    prepaid, 43 (*see also* Prepaid group
        practice)

H

Hampton, J. R., 6
Harvard Community Health Plan,
    xxiv, 58, 61
Hawaii Medical Service Association
    (HMSA), xxiii, 84–85, 92
HealthCare, 168–170
Health care. *See also* Medical care
    doctor-created demand for, 27–28
    impact of regulation in, 112
    main causes of increase in, 16–32
    regional differences in, 28
    regulation of, 113
    sources of spending for, 15

Health Care Financing
    Administration (HCFA), 109
Health care providers, most costly,
    21. *See also* Doctors; Hospitals;
    Physicians
Health care system, decision making
    in, 23
Health Cost Restraint Act of, 1979,
    152
Health, Education, and Welfare,
    Department of (DHEW), 143
Health Incentives Reform Act of 1979
    (HIRA), 152
Health insurance. *See also* Insurance
    coverage
    catastrophic, 157
    consumer vs. job-centered, 115–117
    free market, 78–82
    proposal for national, 115
    regulation of, 77
    as right, 33
    tax credit for, 121–123
Health insurance companies, and
    CCHP, 141
Health Maintenance Organization
    Act of 1973, 76, 143, 146, 153
Health maintenance organizations
    (HMOs), 8
    Blue Cross–Blue Shield sponsored,
        86
    in Carter plan, 169
    definition of, 55
    DHEW responsibility for, 143
    in fair economic competition, 90–91
    in Kennedy health plan, 162
    in Minneapolis–St. Paul, 85–88
    multispecialty group practices
        among, xxiv
    as option, 168
    and physicians' fees, 108
    rapid growth of, 67
    regulation of, 77
    and underservice issue, 68
Health personnel, motivation of, 10.
    See also Doctors; Physicians
Health Plan, Consumer Choice, 36.
    See also Consumer Choice
    Health Plan
Health Planning Act, 156

Health plans. *See also* Insurance plans
    competition among, 20, 82
    criteria for qualified, 126–130
    low option, 128–129
    need for competition among, xxii
    preferred-risk selection for, 80
    SHARE, 86
Health Security Act, 158–161
Health services
    basic, 127–128
    changing sources of funds for, 14–
        15
    lack of fair economic competition
        in, 72–77
    need for standardization of, 81
    regional concentration of, 37–41
    unnecessary, xvii
    variations in per capita use of, 46
Heart attack patients, hospital stay
        for, 46–47
Heart-lung machine, 29
Hellinger, Fred, 102
Henderson, Marie, 143
Hill, J. D., 6
Hinkley, David, 53
Hospital administrators, CCHP for,
        141
Hospital Cost Containment Act, 97,
        99
Hospitalization
    amount of, 25
    and fee structure, 22
    growth in health care spending for,
        14
    for heart attack patients, 47
    incidence of, 6, 44
    major causes of, 8
    and prepaid groups, 60
Hospitals
    average occupancy rates for, 44
    avoidance of regulation, 100
    classifying, 99
    cost containment in, 95–101
    cost reimbursement for, 24–25
    cost of unoccupied beds, 44
    owned by prepaid group practices,
        60
    relationship between volume and
        death rate in, 39

and standard for community bed
        needs, 103–104
Hospital stays
    excessive, 54
    for heart attack patients, 46
Hospital use
    and cost control, xxiii
    and primary care networks, 65–66
Hospital visits, physician's revenue
        for, 22
Hsiao, William, 83
Hutter, Adolph, 46
Hysterectomy, variation in rates of,
        46

I

Identification card, health plan, 130
Immigration laws, 27
Incentives
    for delivery system reform, 118
    financial, 9–10
Income distribution
    and access to medical care, 81
    and demand for health care
        services, 15
Indians, American, financing health
        care for, 131–132
Indicators, health, 7
Individual practice associations
        (*IPAs*), 61–64
    advantages of, 62
    cost control offered by, 76
    disadvantages of, 66
    marketing of, 63–64
Information cost, 81
Information disclosure, 129–130
Inpatient day, 5
Institutionalization, alternatives to, 53
Insurance companies, alternative
        delivery systems developed
        by, 155
Insurance coverage
    casualty, 10–11
    continuity of, 149–150
    duplicate private, 17–18
    free-choice-of-doctor, 26, 77
    and free riders, 78–80

government, 36 (*see also* National health insurance)
growth of, 17–19
impact of, 17–19
impact of tax laws on, 19–21
and information costs, 81
job- vs. consumer-centered, 170
in Kennedy health plan, 162
major risk, 33–35
"low option," 8
mandated employer-provided, 167–170
minimum required standard for, 149
principles of, xviii
rising costs of, xvi
Intensive-care units, 29
Internal Revenue Code, 116, 145
Interstate Commerce Commission, 111
InterStudy, 3
IPAs. *See* Individual practice associations

K

Kaiser-Permanente Medical Care Program, xxiii, xxiv, 43, 58, 68, 75, 90
in Hawaii, 84–85
and hospital beds per capita, 44
Kennedy, Edward M., 55, 135, 157, 171
Kennedy-Mills bill, 158
Kennedy plans, 158–167
Health Care for All Americans, 161
Health Security, 158–161
new, 161
Keynes, John Maynard, 154, 156
Koretz, Daniel, 109
Kramer, Marcia, 27

L

Labor, and health benefits, 19
Lahey Clinic, xxiv
Lee, Philip R., 7

Legislation, health care
Comprehensive National Health Insurance Act of, 1974, 158, 167–170
Health Cost Restraint Act of 1979, 152
Health Incentives Reform Act, 152
Health Maintenance Organization Act of 1973, 76, 143, 146, 153
Health Planning Act, 156
Health Security Act, 158–161
Hospital Cost Containment Act, 97, 99
Kennedy plans, 158–167
National Health Planning and Resources Development Act of 1974, xx, 102, 159
Social Security Act, Title 18, 17
Lembcke, Paul, 7, 46
Lichtner, S., 7
Long, Russell, 157
Luft, Harold, 39, 41, 58, 63, 92
Lunch club analogy, 17

M

McCarthy, Eugene G., 47
McClure, Walter, 3, 56, 57, 88
McDermott, W. V., 53
McNerney, Walter J., 115
Major Risk Insurance, 33–35
objections to, 35
and supplemental private insurance, 35
Malpractice suit, fear of, 32
Mammography, 2
and false-positive rate, 49–50
frequency of, 50
Management, and health benefits, 19
Market economies, advantages of, 112
Maternity, and cost containment, 41
Mather, H. G., 6, 7
May, Joel, 114
Medicaid, 1. *See also* National health insurance
as contributor to New York's financial crisis, 98

Medicaid (*cont.*)
  coverage provided by, 77
  eligibility criteria for, xvi, 18
  inefficiency of, xxii
  limitations of, 75
  and physicians' fees, 105
  size of, 17
  sources of funds for, 19
  as third-party payor, 16
Medical care. *See also* Health care
  amount of, 6–8
  cost-effectiveness analysis in, 165
  and financial incentives, 9–10
  free, 9
  and growth in insurance coverage,
      15
  home vs. hospital, 53
  and longevity, xvi
  measuring quality of, 50–51
  misconceptions about, 1–8
  nature of, xviii
  necessary vs. unnecessary, 11
  organized system for, 67–68
  as public utility, 1
  quality of, 5
  and quality of life, xix, 6
  as right, 12
  science vs. art of, 4
  as standard product, 5
  timing need for, 8
  uncertainty associated with, 2
Medicare, 1
  in CCHP, 124–126
  and cost reimbursement, 76
  coverage for kidney failure, 29
  vs. FEHBP, 83
  fee-screening of, 26
  freedom of choice in, 150
  hospital classification of, 99
  inefficiency of, xxii
  limitations of, 75
  "more vs. better," 6
  and physicians' fees, 105
  and prepaid group practice, 59
  and reasonable charges, 26
  and rising health care costs, xvi
  size of, 17
  sources of funds for, 19
  as third-party payor, 16

Medicine
  as art, 110
  "company store," 21
  "defensive," 16, 32
  "flat-of-the-curve," 45–51
  history of, 51
  "Medi-gap policies," 35
Migrants, financing health care for,
      131–132
Military Health Services System, 131
Mills, Wilbur, 158, 171
Minneapolis–St. Paul, competing
      HMOs in, xxiii, 85–88
Mitchell, J. R. A., 6
Monopoly, IPA-caused, 63–64
Monsma, George, Jr., 10
Multiple choice, principle of, xxii, 71
Myocardial infarction, 6, 7
  early hospital discharge after, 46
  hospitalization for, 47

N

National Health Board, 161, 163, 164
National Health Insurance
  cost estimates for, 135
  government as universal third-
      party payor, 170
  Kennedy plans for, 158–167
  mandated employer-provided
      insurance for, 167–170
  models for, 157
National Health Plan, Carter
      administration's, 105
National Health Planning and
      Resources Development Act of
      1974, xx, 102, 159
Neurosurgery, physician supply in,
      43
Neutra, Raymond, 48
New Mexico Experimental Medical
      Care Review Organization, 109
New York, hospital-rate controls in,
      98–99
Nicollet-Eitel Health Plan, 86
Nixon administration, xx, 55, 105–
      106, 108, 115

health plan proposal of, 167–168, 170

wage and price controls of, 95

Noll, Roger, 111

Nonenrollers, financing health care for, 131–132

Nonprofit institutions, and health tax credits, 146

Nursing home care, growth in health care spending for, 14

O

Office visits, 5
  number of, 25
  physician's revenue for, 22
  unnecessary, 31–32

Open-heart surgery, 29, 37–41

Operations
  and cost efficiency, 38
  discarded, 5
  necessity for, 3
  relationship between volume and death rate, 39–41
  variations in rates of, 48

Ophthalmology, physician supply in, 43

Outpatient services, costs for, 32

P

Palo Alto Medical Clinic, 9–10, 61

Pap smear, frequency of, 50

Patients. *See also* Consumers; Hospitalization
  heart attack, 96
  and prepaid group practice plan, 61

Payment
  fee-for-service, 9, 10, 21–23, 43
  inefficiency associated with, 17
  per capita, 23

PCN. *See* Primary care network

Peer review, in individual practice association, 63

Pettigrew, Ann, 41

Pflanz, M., 7

Photocoagulation, 3

Physicians. *See also* Doctors
  control over medical expenditures, 23
  controls on fees of, 105–108
  in group practice, 60
  incentives for, 10
  motivation of, 10
  in prepaid group practice, 58
  and supply and demand, 27
  supply of, 42

Physicians Association of Clackamas County, 62

Physicians' fees. *See also* Fee structure
  and CPI, 106
  government controls on, 108
  and Economic Stabilization Program, 106
  and HMOs, 108
  and Medicaid/Medicare, 105
  in national health insurance, 171

Physicians Health Plan (Minnesota), 62, 63

Physicians Health Plan, of Hennepin County Medical Society, 87

Piecework system, xvii

Pigou, A. C., 70

Political-reward system, 161

Poor
  CCHP and, 139, 142
  and health plan competition, 88
  response to needs of, 89
  subsidy of medical care for, 81
  vouchers for, 123–124

Population, matching resources to needs of, 44, 57

Preferred-risk selection, 80, 153

Premiums. *See also* Insurance coverage
  "earnings-based," 135
  experience rating for, 25
  HMO, 59
  increases in, 18
  under Kennedy plan, 163
  mandatory, 79, 82, 122
  rating by market area, 128
  "wage-related," 163, 166

Prepaid group practice, 10, 57–61
  costs compared with Medicare, 76

Prepaid group practice (*cont.*)
  effectiveness of, 58
  in fair economic competition, 92
  and high-mobility population, 61
  under Kennedy health plan, 162
  and medical costs, xix
  principles of, 58
  and quality control, 60
  Medicaid-oriented, 68
  and use of services, 9
Price controls
  as cost reimbursement, 100
  on hospitals, 95
  and physician fees, 106
  proposals for, xx
Primary care network (PCN), 64
  and hospital use, 65–66
Professional Standards Review
    Organizations (PSROs), xx, 4,
    156
  creation of, 108–109
  failure of, 110
  in Kennedy health plan, 163
Project Health of Multnomah
    County, Oregon, 88–89
Public funds, equitable distribution
    of, 117
Public policy, toward delivery-system
    reform, 133–134
Public-utility approach, to medical
    care financing, 5
Puget Sound, Group Health
    Cooperative of, 44, 58, 65, 68,
    124

Q

Quality of care
  consumer vs. provider concept of,
    50–51
  and economy, xix
  and group practice, 60
Quality of life, and medical care, 6

R

Ramsey Health Plan, 86
Randomized clinical trial (RCT), 4

Reform, need for, xxi–xxv. *See also*
    Delivery systems
Regional centers
  for maternity centers, 41
  for open-heart surgery, 40
Regulation
  and certificates of need, 101–105
  and competition, xx, xxi–xxii, 101–
    113
  and consumer costs, 111
  control on physicians' fees, 105–108
  definition for, 71
  vs. economic incentives, 93–95
  limitations of, xxi
  procompetitive, 94
  proposals for, xx
Reinhardt, Uwe, 28
Renal dialysis, 29
Resources, and needs of population,
    42–44
Retainer fee, 23
Retina, detached, 3
Rettig, Richard, 30
Ribicoff, Abraham, 157
Ross-Loos, 58
Routine cost, 24
Roy, William R., 55
Ruddock, Andrew, 83
Rural areas, and CCHP, 140
Russell, Louise, 29

S

SAFECO Life Insurance Co. of
    Seattle, 64, 65, 92, 121
St. Louis Park Medical Center, 61,
    86, 88
St. Paul, Minnesota, Group Health
    Plan of, 58
Salkever, David, 102
San Francisco, physician supply in,
    43
San Joaquin Foundation for Medical
    Care, 62
Schultze, Charles, 70–71, 113
Schweiker, Richard, 152
Science, medical care as, 9
Scitovsky, Anne, 9, 10

Securities and Exchange
Commission, 93
Services. *See* Health services
SHARE Health Plan, 86
Sickness, nature of, 80
Silverman, Milton, 8
Sloan, Frank, 96, 98, 102
Smith, Adam, 70
Social Security Act, Title 18 of, 17
Somers, Anne, 114
Somers, Herman, 114
Specialists, vs. general practitioners,
xvii
Spending, health care. *See also*
Expenditures
causes of increased, xvii–xxi, 16–32
growth of, xv–xvii, 13–14
Standards
in benefits plans, 149–150
best-treatment, 4
professional review organizations
for, xx, 4, 108–109, 110, 156,
163
for services, 81
for treatment, 4
State government
and CCHP financing and
administration, 130
as third-party payor, 25
State Health Boards, 161, 162
State Negotiating Group, 164
Statistics, and health costs projection,
124
Steinwald, Bruce, 96, 98, 102
Stockman, David, 152
Subsidies, government. *See also* Tax
credits
actuarial costs-based, 119–120
fixed-dollar, 71–72
Surgery
coronary artery bypass graft, 5, 52
evaluation of, 52
outpatient, 53
regional concentration of, 37–41
"same day," 53
second opinions for, 47–48
"unnecessary," 47
variation in per capita use of, 46
"Swiss cheese policies," 128

T

Taxation, reduction of, 16
Tax credits, 121–123
and CCHP, 136
for employer contributions, 150–
151
and nonprofit employers, 146
Tax laws
effect on medical costs, 75
impact of, 19–21, 117–118
inefficiency of, xxii
Tax subsidies, 79, 82. *See also*
Subsidies
Taylor, Amy, 18
Technological advances, 28–31
controlling, 51–53
and health care costs, 21–22
international character of, 31
and quality of life, 15
Technology
controlled introduction of, 51–53
cost-reducing, 30
Third-party payors, xvii, 16
government as universal, 158, 170–
172
and hospital costs, 23
Medicaid/Medicare, 16
passive role of, 25–27
Thompson, Alvin, 22
Tonsillectomy, variation in rates of,
46
"Top-down budgeting," 160, 161
Treatment
standard, 4
variation in, 2–4
Twin Cities Health Care
Development Project, 87

U

Ullman, Al, 151, 152, 156
Underworld, financing health care
for, 131–132
Unions. *See also* Employers
and CCHP, 142
and health benefits, 19

United Kingdom, home vs. hospital
care studies in, 53
United States, physician supply in,
43
Utilization Review, 108–110

V

Vayda, Eugene, 172
Veterans, financing health care for,
131–132
Veterans Administration (VA), health
care system of, xxi, 131–132,
160
Voucher system, 123–124
and CCHP, 136

W

Washington, D.C., Group Health
Association of, 58
Waste, 54
Wennberg, John, 46
West Bay Health System Agency, of
San Francisco, 104–105
Wilson, Lawrence, 98
Wisconsin Physicians Service Health
Maintenance Program, 64
Workers, in CCHP, 141–142. *See also*
Employees; Unions